MW00574052

THE MARIJUANA JOURNAL

THE
MARIJUANA
JOURNAL

A Notebook and Diary to Record (and Remember) Your Favorite Cannabis Strains, Edibles, Recipes, Brilliant Ideas, and Hazy Experiences

HERBIE A. STONER

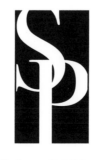

Skyhorse Publishing

Skyhorse Publishing books may be purchased in bulk at special discounts for sales promotion, corporate gifts, fund-raising, or educational purposes. Special editions can also be created to specifications. For details, contact the Special Sales Department, Skyhorse Publishing, 307 West 36th Street, 11th Floor, New York, NY 10018 or info@skyhorsepublishing.com.

Skyhorse® and Skyhorse Publishing® are registered trademarks of Skyhorse Publishing, Inc.®, a Delaware corporation.

Visit our website at www.skyhorsepublishing.com.

10 9 8 7 6 5 4 3 2 1

Library of Congress Cataloging-in-Publication Data is available on file.

Cover design by Kai Texel
Cover image credit: Getty Images

Print ISBN: 978-1-5107-6992-2
Ebook ISBN: 978-1-5107-7191-8

Printed in China

CONTENTS

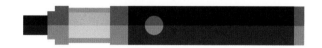

INTRODUCTION

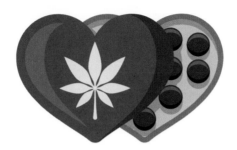

"Ugh, what was the name of that strain again? The good one? That one we smoked last time?"

For those of you who enjoy smoking, vaping, ingesting, or any other method of taking cannabis, this is most likely a thought you've had. Nothing is worse than enjoying some herb and completely forgetting the name or the strain.

Even so, when visiting your neighborhood budtender, it may be frustrting trying to remember which of their choices you already had, and if you liked them or not.

Well, fear not!

The goal of *The Marijuana Journal* is just that: a method to "chronic"le each and every strain you've tried, what your thoughts were, how if affected you, and any additional notes you feel worth including.

Cannabis affects us all differently, so creating a journal where you can personally add your thoughts seemed like a no-brainer. While many of us rely on websites like Leafly and what we've read in *High Times* magazine, nobody knows better than you how your body reacts to a specific strain.

As more states and countries realize that marijuana is not the enemy, and even more realizing their medicinal properties, users will have more information to absorb then they know what to do with! So why spend all that time researching and trying to remember how you felt when you can log it in this journal for future reference.

Because when you open *The Marijuana Journal* and read that you had a negative trip from OG Kush but really enjoyed Blue Dream, you will be able to not only purchase the strains you enjoyed most, but have a better expectation as to how you body will respond.

While it goes without saying, you should always be smart and safe when imbibing. Do not drive, operate machinery, or do anything that you wouldn't be comfortable with unless sober. Be smart. Remember: the cannabis community is one of love and affection. Make sure to *never* do anything that might put yourself—or others—in harms way. That goes for the environment as well!

We hope you enjoy this journal and use it to improve your sessions, however you choose to imbibe.

Your friendly pothead,
Herbie A. Stoner

THE MARIJUANA JOURNAL

STRAIN ENTRIES

Strain Name: _____

Date: _____

Time taken: _____ Time it took to feel effects: _____

Strain Type: □ Sativa   □ Indica   □ Hybrid   □ Not sure

Medium of Consumption: □ Flower   □ Edible   □ Concentrate   □ Other _____

Method: □ Smoke   □ Vape   □ Ingest   □ Other _____

Potency:
(Circle one)

🍁 🍁 🍁 🍁 🍁 🍁 🍁 🍁 🍁 🍁
1   2   3   4   5   6   7   8   9   10

THC % _____ CBD % _____ CBN % _____ Other % _____

Appearance and Taste

Aroma: _____

Color: _____

Flavor Notes: _____

Positive Effects:

□ **Creative**   □ **Happy**   □ **Energetic**   □ **Euphoric**   □ **Relaxed**   □ **Talkative**

□ **Uplifted**   □ **Zen**   □ **Other:** _____

Negative Effects:

□ **Anxiety**   □ **Cotton mouth**   □ **Couch lock**   □ **Dizziness**   □ **Dry eyes**

□ **Memory Problems**   □ **Paranoid**   □ **Other:** _____

Helps with:

□ **General Pain**   □ **Back Pain**   □ **Anxiety**   □ **Depression**   □ **Concentration**

□ **Sleep Problems**   □ **Other:** _____

Would try again?

□ Yes   □ No

Overall Rating:
(Circle one)

🍁 🍁 🍁 🍁 🍁 🍁 🍁 🍁 🍁 🍁
1   2   3   4   5   6   7   8   9   10

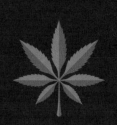

"Alcohol and marijuana, if used in moderation, plus loud, usually low-class music, make stress and boredom infinitely more bearable."
—Kurt Vonnegut

Notes:

Strain Name: _____

Date: _____

Time taken: _____ Time it took to feel effects: _____

Strain Type: □ Sativa   □ Indica   □ Hybrid   □ Not sure

Medium of Consumption: □ Flower   □ Edible   □ Concentrate   □ Other _____

Method: □ Smoke   □ Vape   □ Ingest   □ Other _____

Potency:
(Circle one)
1   2   3   4   5   6   7   8   9   10

THC % _____ CBD % _____ CBN % _____ Other % _____

Appearance and Taste

Aroma: _____

Color: _____

Flavor Notes: _____

Positive Effects:

□ **Creative**   □ **Happy**   □ **Energetic**   □ **Euphoric**   □ **Relaxed**   □ **Talkative**

□ **Uplifted**   □ **Zen**   □ **Other:** _____

Negative Effects:

□ **Anxiety**   □ **Cotton mouth**   □ **Couch lock**   □ **Dizziness**   □ **Dry eyes**

□ **Memory Problems**   □ **Paranoid**   □ **Other:** _____

Helps with:

□ **General Pain**   □ **Back Pain**   □ **Anxiety**   □ **Depression**   □ **Concentration**

□ **Sleep Problems**   □ **Other:** _____

Would try again?

□ Yes   □ No

Overall Rating:
(Circle one)
1   2   3   4   5   6   7   8   9   10

Notes:

_____

_____

_____

_____

_____

_____

_____

_____

_____

_____

_____

_____

_____

_____

Tip: Edibles are ingested through your saliva! So instead of swallowing that brownie whole, chew the ever-living crap out of it. That'll get you a lot higher than just scarfing it down.

Strain Name: _____

Date: _____

Time taken: _____ Time it took to feel effects: _____

Strain Type: □ Sativa   □ Indica   □ Hybrid   □ Not sure

Medium of Consumption: □ Flower   □ Edible   □ Concentrate   □ Other _____

Method: □ Smoke   □ Vape   □ Ingest   □ Other _____

Potency:
(Circle one)   1   2   3   4   5   6   7   8   9   10

THC % _____ CBD % _____ CBN % _____ Other % _____

Appearance and Taste

Aroma: _____

Color: _____

Flavor Notes: _____

Positive Effects:

□ Creative   □ Happy   □ Energetic   □ Euphoric   □ Relaxed   □ Talkative

□ Uplifted   □ Zen   □ Other: _____

Negative Effects:

□ Anxiety   □ Cotton mouth   □ Couch lock   □ Dizziness   □ Dry eyes

□ Memory Problems   □ Paranoid   □ Other: _____

Helps with:

□ General Pain   □ Back Pain   □ Anxiety   □ Depression   □ Concentration

□ Sleep Problems   □ Other: _____

Would try again?

□ Yes   □ No

Overall Rating:
(Circle one)   1   2   3   4   5   6   7   8   9   10

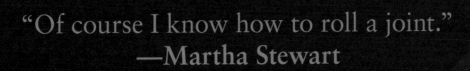 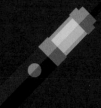

"Of course I know how to roll a joint."
—Martha Stewart

Notes:

Strain Name: _____

Date: _____

Time taken: _____ Time it took to feel effects: _____

Strain Type: ☐ Sativa ☐ Indica ☐ Hybrid ☐ Not sure

Medium of Consumption: ☐ Flower ☐ Edible ☐ Concentrate ☐ Other _____

Method: ☐ Smoke ☐ Vape ☐ Ingest ☐ Other _____

Potency:
(Circle one)

| 1 | 2 | 3 | 4 | 5 | 6 | 7 | 8 | 9 | 10 |

THC % _____ CBD % _____ CBN % _____ Other % _____

Appearance and Taste

Aroma: _____

Color: _____

Flavor Notes: _____

Positive Effects:

☐ Creative ☐ Happy ☐ Energetic ☐ Euphoric ☐ Relaxed ☐ Talkative

☐ Uplifted ☐ Zen ☐ Other: _____

Negative Effects:

☐ Anxiety ☐ Cotton mouth ☐ Couch lock ☐ Dizziness ☐ Dry eyes

☐ Memory Problems ☐ Paranoid ☐ Other: _____

Helps with:

☐ General Pain ☐ Back Pain ☐ Anxiety ☐ Depression ☐ Concentration

☐ Sleep Problems ☐ Other: _____

Would try again?

☐ Yes ☐ No

Overall Rating:
(Circle one)

| 1 | 2 | 3 | 4 | 5 | 6 | 7 | 8 | 9 | 10 |

Tip: Proceed with extreme caution when partaking in edibles. Wait the extra hour and see how you feel before scarfing down that second half of the brownie.

Notes:

Strain Name: _____

Date: _____

Time taken:_____ Time it took to feel effects: _____

Strain Type: ☐ Sativa   ☐ Indica   ☐ Hybrid   ☐ Not sure

Medium of Consumption: ☐ Flower   ☐ Edible   ☐ Concentrate   ☐ Other _____

Method: ☐ Smoke   ☐ Vape   ☐ Ingest   ☐ Other _____

Potency:
(Circle one)   🍁 1   🍁 2   🍁 3   🍁 4   🍁 5   🍁 6   🍁 7   🍁 8   🍁 9   🍁 10

THC % _____ CBD % _____ CBN % _____ Other % _____

Appearance and Taste

Aroma: _____

Color: _____

Flavor Notes: _____

Positive Effects:

☐ Creative   ☐ Happy   ☐ Energetic   ☐ Euphoric   ☐ Relaxed   ☐ Talkative

☐ Uplifted   ☐ Zen   ☐ Other: _____

Negative Effects:

☐ Anxiety   ☐ Cotton mouth   ☐ Couch lock   ☐ Dizziness   ☐ Dry eyes

☐ Memory Problems   ☐ Paranoid   ☐ Other: _____

Helps with:

☐ General Pain   ☐ Back Pain   ☐ Anxiety   ☐ Depression   ☐ Concentration

☐ Sleep Problems   ☐ Other: _____

Would try again?

☐ Yes   ☐ No

Overall Rating:
(Circle one)   🍁 1   🍁 2   🍁 3   🍁 4   🍁 5   🍁 6   🍁 7   🍁 8   🍁 9   🍁 10

Notes:

Strain Name: _____

Date: _____

Time taken: _____ Time it took to feel effects: _____

Strain Type: □ Sativa □ Indica □ Hybrid □ Not sure

Medium of Consumption: □ Flower □ Edible □ Concentrate □ Other _____

Method: □ Smoke □ Vape □ Ingest □ Other _____

Potency:
(Circle one)   🍁 🍁 🍁 🍁 🍁 🍁 🍁 🍁 🍁 🍁
                 1   2   3   4   5   6   7   8   9   10

THC % _____ CBD % _____ CBN % _____ Other % _____

Appearance and Taste

Aroma: _____

Color: _____

Flavor Notes: _____

Positive Effects:

□ Creative □ Happy □ Energetic □ Euphoric □ Relaxed □ Talkative

□ Uplifted □ Zen □ Other: _____

Negative Effects:

□ Anxiety □ Cotton mouth □ Couch lock □ Dizziness □ Dry eyes

□ Memory Problems □ Paranoid □ Other: _____

Helps with:

□ General Pain □ Back Pain □ Anxiety □ Depression □ Concentration

□ Sleep Problems □ Other: _____

Would try again?

□ Yes □ No

Overall Rating:
(Circle one)   🍁 🍁 🍁 🍁 🍁 🍁 🍁 🍁 🍁 🍁
                 1   2   3   4   5   6   7   8   9   10

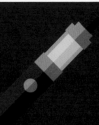

Tip: While the old adage is that Indica will put you in da couch, that is not always true. Make sure to do your own research on any strain so that you know how your body and mind will react.

Notes:

Strain Name: _____

Date: _____

Time taken: _____   Time it took to feel effects: _____

Strain Type: ☐ Sativa   ☐ Indica   ☐ Hybrid   ☐ Not sure

Medium of Consumption: ☐ Flower   ☐ Edible   ☐ Concentrate   ☐ Other _____

Method: ☐ Smoke   ☐ Vape   ☐ Ingest   ☐ Other _____

Potency:
(Circle one)

🍁 🍁 🍁 🍁 🍁 🍁 🍁 🍁 🍁 🍁
1   2   3   4   5   6   7   8   9   10

THC % _____   CBD % _____   CBN % _____   Other % _____

Appearance and Taste

Aroma: _____

Color: _____

Flavor Notes: _____

Positive Effects:

☐ Creative   ☐ Happy   ☐ Energetic   ☐ Euphoric   ☐ Relaxed   ☐ Talkative

☐ Uplifted   ☐ Zen   ☐ Other: _____

Negative Effects:

☐ Anxiety   ☐ Cotton mouth   ☐ Couch lock   ☐ Dizziness   ☐ Dry eyes

☐ Memory Problems   ☐ Paranoid   ☐ Other: _____

Helps with:

☐ General Pain   ☐ Back Pain   ☐ Anxiety   ☐ Depression   ☐ Concentration

☐ Sleep Problems   ☐ Other: _____

Would try again?

☐ Yes   ☐ No

Overall Rating:
(Circle one)

🍁 🍁 🍁 🍁 🍁 🍁 🍁 🍁 🍁 🍁
1   2   3   4   5   6   7   8   9   10

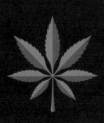

"If more people were stoned there would be less violence in the world." —Tommy Chong

Notes:

_____

_____

_____

_____

_____

_____

_____

_____

_____

_____

_____

_____

_____

_____

_____

_____

_____

Strain Name: _____

Date: _____

Time taken: _____ Time it took to feel effects: _____

Strain Type: □ Sativa □ Indica □ Hybrid □ Not sure

Medium of Consumption: □ Flower □ Edible □ Concentrate □ Other _____

Method: □ Smoke □ Vape □ Ingest □ Other _____

Potency:
(Circle one)
1   2   3   4   5   6   7   8   9   10

THC % _____ CBD % _____ CBN % _____ Other % _____

Appearance and Taste

Aroma: _____

Color: _____

Flavor Notes: _____

Positive Effects:

□ **Creative** □ **Happy** □ **Energetic** □ **Euphoric** □ **Relaxed** □ **Talkative**

□ **Uplifted** □ **Zen** □ **Other:** _____

Negative Effects:

□ **Anxiety** □ **Cotton mouth** □ **Couch lock** □ **Dizziness** □ **Dry eyes**

□ **Memory Problems** □ **Paranoid** □ **Other:** _____

Helps with:

□ **General Pain** □ **Back Pain** □ **Anxiety** □ **Depression** □ **Concentration**

□ **Sleep Problems** □ **Other:** _____

Would try again?

□ Yes □ No

Overall Rating:
(Circle one)
1   2   3   4   5   6   7   8   9   10

Notes:

_____

_____

_____

_____

_____

_____

_____

_____

_____

_____

_____

_____

_____

_____

_____

_____

Tip: "When smoking cannabis, consider making it a slow, deliberate affair. Take a couple long hits off the pipe and then kick back for a few. It can take up to around 15 minutes for you to feel the high from smoking weed, and by then, you may realize that those two hits got you plenty high, without having to burn the other half of the bowl." (PlantsandPrescriptions.com)

Strain Name: _____

Date: _____

Time taken: _____ Time it took to feel effects: _____

Strain Type: □ Sativa □ Indica □ Hybrid □ Not sure

Medium of Consumption: □ Flower □ Edible □ Concentrate □ Other _____

Method: □ Smoke □ Vape □ Ingest □ Other _____

Potency:
(Circle one)

🌿 🌿 🌿 🌿 🌿 🌿 🌿 🌿 🌿 🌿
1   2   3   4   5   6   7   8   9   10

THC % _____ CBD % _____ CBN % _____ Other % _____

Appearance and Taste

Aroma: _____

Color: _____

Flavor Notes: _____

Positive Effects:

□ **Creative** □ **Happy** □ **Energetic** □ **Euphoric** □ **Relaxed** □ **Talkative**

□ **Uplifted** □ **Zen** □ **Other:** _____

Negative Effects:

□ **Anxiety** □ **Cotton mouth** □ **Couch lock** □ **Dizziness** □ **Dry eyes**

□ **Memory Problems** □ **Paranoid** □ **Other:** _____

Helps with:

□ **General Pain** □ **Back Pain** □ **Anxiety** □ **Depression** □ **Concentration**

□ **Sleep Problems** □ **Other:** _____

Would try again?

□ Yes □ No

Overall Rating:
(Circle one)

🌿 🌿 🌿 🌿 🌿 🌿 🌿 🌿 🌿 🌿
1   2   3   4   5   6   7   8   9   10

> "When you smoke the herb,
> it reveals you to yourself."
> —Bob Marley

Notes:

_____

_____

_____

_____

_____

_____

_____

_____

_____

_____

_____

_____

_____

_____

_____

_____

_____

_____

Strain Name: _____

Date: _____

Time taken: _____ Time it took to feel effects: _____

Strain Type: □ Sativa   □ Indica   □ Hybrid   □ Not sure

Medium of Consumption: □ Flower   □ Edible   □ Concentrate   □ Other _____

Method: □ Smoke   □ Vape   □ Ingest   □ Other _____

Potency:
(Circle one)

1   2   3   4   5   6   7   8   9   10

THC % _____ CBD % _____ CBN % _____ Other % _____

Appearance and Taste

Aroma: _____

Color: _____

Flavor Notes: _____

Positive Effects:

□ Creative   □ Happy   □ Energetic   □ Euphoric   □ Relaxed   □ Talkative

□ Uplifted   □ Zen   □ Other: _____

Negative Effects:

□ Anxiety   □ Cotton mouth   □ Couch lock   □ Dizziness   □ Dry eyes

□ Memory Problems   □ Paranoid   □ Other: _____

Helps with:

□ General Pain   □ Back Pain   □ Anxiety   □ Depression   □ Concentration

□ Sleep Problems   □ Other: _____

Would try again?

□ Yes   □ No

Overall Rating:
(Circle one)

1   2   3   4   5   6   7   8   9   10

Tip: Make sure to keep water and eye drops on hand, as dry mouth and dry eyes are common side effects!

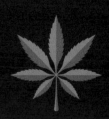

Notes:

_____

_____

_____

_____

_____

_____

_____

_____

_____

_____

_____

_____

_____

_____

_____

Strain Name: _____

Date: _____

Time taken: _____ Time it took to feel effects: _____

Strain Type: □ Sativa   □ Indica   □ Hybrid   □ Not sure

Medium of Consumption: □ Flower   □ Edible   □ Concentrate   □ Other _____

Method: □ Smoke   □ Vape   □ Ingest   □ Other _____

Potency:
(Circle one)

🌿 🌿 🌿 🌿 🌿 🌿 🌿 🌿 🌿 🌿
1   2   3   4   5   6   7   8   9   10

THC % _____ CBD % _____ CBN % _____ Other % _____

Appearance and Taste

Aroma: _____

Color: _____

Flavor Notes: _____

Positive Effects:

□ **Creative**   □ **Happy**   □ **Energetic**   □ **Euphoric**   □ **Relaxed**   □ **Talkative**

□ **Uplifted**   □ **Zen**   □ **Other:** _____

Negative Effects:

□ **Anxiety**   □ **Cotton mouth**   □ **Couch lock**   □ **Dizziness**   □ **Dry eyes**

□ **Memory Problems**   □ **Paranoid**   □ **Other:** _____

Helps with:

□ **General Pain**   □ **Back Pain**   □ **Anxiety**   □ **Depression**   □ **Concentration**

□ **Sleep Problems**   □ **Other:** _____

Would try again?

□ **Yes**   □ **No**

Overall Rating:
(Circle one)

🌿 🌿 🌿 🌿 🌿 🌿 🌿 🌿 🌿 🌿
1   2   3   4   5   6   7   8   9   10

Notes:

_____

_____

_____

_____

_____

_____

_____

_____

_____

_____

_____

_____

_____

_____

_____

"When I was a kid I inhaled frequently.
That was the point."
—President Barack Obama

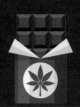

Strain Name: _____

Date: _____

Time taken: _____ Time it took to feel effects: _____

Strain Type: ☐ Sativa ☐ Indica ☐ Hybrid ☐ Not sure

Medium of Consumption: ☐ Flower ☐ Edible ☐ Concentrate ☐ Other _____

Method: ☐ Smoke ☐ Vape ☐ Ingest ☐ Other _____

Potency:
(Circle one)
1   2   3   4   5   6   7   8   9   10

THC % _____ CBD % _____ CBN % _____ Other % _____

Appearance and Taste

Aroma: _____

Color: _____

Flavor Notes: _____

Positive Effects:

☐ Creative ☐ Happy ☐ Energetic ☐ Euphoric ☐ Relaxed ☐ Talkative

☐ Uplifted ☐ Zen ☐ Other: _____

Negative Effects:

☐ Anxiety ☐ Cotton mouth ☐ Couch lock ☐ Dizziness ☐ Dry eyes

☐ Memory Problems ☐ Paranoid ☐ Other: _____

Helps with:

☐ General Pain ☐ Back Pain ☐ Anxiety ☐ Depression ☐ Concentration

☐ Sleep Problems ☐ Other: _____

Would try again?

☐ Yes ☐ No

Overall Rating:
(Circle one)
1   2   3   4   5   6   7   8   9   10

Tip: "Eating mangos is one tested and trusted hack that can help in your quest to stay higher longer. Mangoes contain myrcene, which is a terpene also found in cannabis." (Ally Hilbert, Elevate Holistics)

Notes:

_____

_____

_____

_____

_____

_____

_____

_____

_____

_____

_____

_____

_____

_____

_____

_____

Strain Name: _____

Date: _____

Time taken: _____ Time it took to feel effects: _____

Strain Type: □ Sativa □ Indica □ Hybrid □ Not sure

Medium of Consumption: □ Flower □ Edible □ Concentrate □ Other _____

Method: □ Smoke □ Vape □ Ingest □ Other _____

Potency:
(Circle one)

🍁 🍁 🍁 🍁 🍁 🍁 🍁 🍁 🍁 🍁
1   2   3   4   5   6   7   8   9   10

THC % _____ CBD % _____ CBN % _____ Other % _____

Appearance and Taste

Aroma: _____

Color: _____

Flavor Notes: _____

Positive Effects:

□ Creative   □ Happy   □ Energetic   □ Euphoric   □ Relaxed   □ Talkative

□ Uplifted   □ Zen   □ Other: _____

Negative Effects:

□ Anxiety   □ Cotton mouth   □ Couch lock   □ Dizziness   □ Dry eyes

□ Memory Problems   □ Paranoid   □ Other: _____

Helps with:

□ General Pain   □ Back Pain   □ Anxiety   □ Depression   □ Concentration

□ Sleep Problems   □ Other: _____

Would try again?

□ Yes   □ No

Overall Rating:
(Circle one)

🍁 🍁 🍁 🍁 🍁 🍁 🍁 🍁 🍁 🍁
1   2   3   4   5   6   7   8   9   10

> "If you substitute marijuana for tobacco and alcohol, you'll add eight to twenty-four years to your life."
> —Jack Herer

Notes:

_____

_____

_____

_____

_____

_____

_____

_____

_____

_____

_____

_____

_____

_____

_____

_____

_____

Strain Name: _____

Date: _____

Time taken: _____ Time it took to feel effects: _____

Strain Type: □ Sativa □ Indica □ Hybrid □ Not sure

Medium of Consumption: □ Flower □ Edible □ Concentrate □ Other _____

Method: □ Smoke □ Vape □ Ingest □ Other _____

Potency:
(Circle one)
1 2 3 4 5 6 7 8 9 10

THC % _____ CBD % _____ CBN % _____ Other % _____

Appearance and Taste

Aroma: _____

Color: _____

Flavor Notes: _____

Positive Effects:

□ Creative □ Happy □ Energetic □ Euphoric □ Relaxed □ Talkative

□ Uplifted □ Zen □ Other: _____

Negative Effects:

□ Anxiety □ Cotton mouth □ Couch lock □ Dizziness □ Dry eyes

□ Memory Problems □ Paranoid □ Other: _____

Helps with:

□ General Pain □ Back Pain □ Anxiety □ Depression □ Concentration

□ Sleep Problems □ Other: _____

Would try again?

□ Yes □ No

Overall Rating:
(Circle one)
1 2 3 4 5 6 7 8 9 10

Notes:

_____

_____

_____

_____

_____

_____

_____

_____

_____

_____

_____

_____

_____

_____

Tip: When you need to clean your bowl, pipe, bubbler, or bong, look no further than rubbing alcohol and salt! Soaking your piece(s) in Isopropal alcohol and table salt will do wonders. Overnight or 24 hours should do the trick.

Strain Name: _____

Date: _____

Time taken: _____   Time it took to feel effects: _____

Strain Type: □ Sativa   □ Indica   □ Hybrid   □ Not sure

Medium of Consumption: □ Flower   □ Edible   □ Concentrate   □ Other _____

Method: □ Smoke   □ Vape   □ Ingest   □ Other _____

Potency:
(Circle one)
1   2   3   4   5   6   7   8   9   10

THC % _____   CBD % _____   CBN % _____   Other % _____

Appearance and Taste

Aroma: _____

Color: _____

Flavor Notes: _____

Positive Effects:

□ Creative   □ Happy   □ Energetic   □ Euphoric   □ Relaxed   □ Talkative

□ Uplifted   □ Zen   □ Other: _____

Negative Effects:

□ Anxiety   □ Cotton mouth   □ Couch lock   □ Dizziness   □ Dry eyes

□ Memory Problems   □ Paranoid   □ Other: _____

Helps with:

□ General Pain   □ Back Pain   □ Anxiety   □ Depression   □ Concentration

□ Sleep Problems   □ Other: _____

Would try again?

□ Yes   □ No

Overall Rating:
(Circle one)
1   2   3   4   5   6   7   8   9   10

One's condition on marijuana is always existential. One can feel the importance of each moment and how it is changing one. One feels one's being, one becomes aware of the enormous apparatus of nothingness—the hum of a hi-fi set, the emptiness of a pointless interruption, one becomes aware of the war between each of us, how the nothingness in each of us seeks to attack the being of others, how our being in turn is attacked by the nothingness in others." —**Norman Mailer**

Notes:

Strain Name: _____

Date: _____

Time taken: _____   Time it took to feel effects: _____

Strain Type: □ Sativa   □ Indica   □ Hybrid   □ Not sure

Medium of Consumption: □ Flower   □ Edible   □ Concentrate   □ Other _____

Method: □ Smoke   □ Vape   □ Ingest   □ Other _____

Potency:
(Circle one)
1   2   3   4   5   6   7   8   9   10

THC % _____ CBD % _____ CBN % _____ Other % _____

Appearance and Taste

Aroma: _____

Color: _____

Flavor Notes: _____

Positive Effects:

□ **Creative**   □ **Happy**   □ **Energetic**   □ **Euphoric**   □ **Relaxed**   □ **Talkative**

□ **Uplifted**   □ **Zen**   □ **Other:** _____

Negative Effects:

□ **Anxiety**   □ **Cotton mouth**   □ **Couch lock**   □ **Dizziness**   □ **Dry eyes**

□ **Memory Problems**   □ **Paranoid**   □ **Other:** _____

Helps with:

□ **General Pain**   □ **Back Pain**   □ **Anxiety**   □ **Depression**   □ **Concentration**

□ **Sleep Problems**   □ **Other:** _____

Would try again?

□ Yes   □ No

Overall Rating:
(Circle one)
1   2   3   4   5   6   7   8   9   10

Notes:

Strain Name: _____

Date: _____

Time taken: _____   Time it took to feel effects: _____

Strain Type: □ Sativa   □ Indica   □ Hybrid   □ Not sure

Medium of Consumption: □ Flower   □ Edible   □ Concentrate   □ Other _____

Method: □ Smoke   □ Vape   □ Ingest   □ Other _____

Potency:
(Circle one)   1   2   3   4   5   6   7   8   9   10

THC % _____   CBD % _____   CBN % _____   Other % _____

Appearance and Taste

Aroma: _____

Color: _____

Flavor Notes: _____

Positive Effects:

□ Creative   □ Happy   □ Energetic   □ Euphoric   □ Relaxed   □ Talkative

□ Uplifted   □ Zen   □ Other: _____

Negative Effects:

□ Anxiety   □ Cotton mouth   □ Couch lock   □ Dizziness   □ Dry eyes

□ Memory Problems   □ Paranoid   □ Other: _____

Helps with:

□ General Pain   □ Back Pain   □ Anxiety   □ Depression   □ Concentration

□ Sleep Problems   □ Other: _____

Would try again?

□ Yes   □ No

Overall Rating:
(Circle one)   1   2   3   4   5   6   7   8   9   10

Notes:

"I have always loved marijuana. It has been a source of joy and comfort to me for many years. And I still think of it as a basic staple of life, along with beer and ice and grapefruits—and millions of Americans agree with me." —Hunter S. Thompson

Strain Name: _____

Date: _____

Time taken: _____ Time it took to feel effects: _____

Strain Type: □ Sativa □ Indica □ Hybrid □ Not sure

Medium of Consumption: □ Flower □ Edible □ Concentrate □ Other _____

Method: □ Smoke □ Vape □ Ingest □ Other _____

Potency:
(Circle one)
🍁 🍁 🍁 🍁 🍁 🍁 🍁 🍁 🍁 🍁
1   2   3   4   5   6   7   8   9   10

THC % _____ CBD % _____ CBN % _____ Other % _____

Appearance and Taste

Aroma: _____

Color: _____

Flavor Notes: _____

Positive Effects:

□ Creative □ Happy □ Energetic □ Euphoric □ Relaxed □ Talkative

□ Uplifted □ Zen □ Other: _____

Negative Effects:

□ Anxiety □ Cotton mouth □ Couch lock □ Dizziness □ Dry eyes

□ Memory Problems □ Paranoid □ Other: _____

Helps with:

□ General Pain □ Back Pain □ Anxiety □ Depression □ Concentration

□ Sleep Problems □ Other: _____

Would try again?

□ Yes □ No

Overall Rating:
(Circle one)
🍁 🍁 🍁 🍁 🍁 🍁 🍁 🍁 🍁 🍁
1   2   3   4   5   6   7   8   9   10

Tip: We know that you should never go food shopping when hungry. Well, the same applies to being stoned! Unless you're on a munchies run for friends (and didn't drive!), make sure to avoid buying a dozen bags of Doritos and three pints of Ben & Jerry's.

Notes:

Strain Name: _____

Date: _____

Time taken: _____ Time it took to feel effects: _____

Strain Type: ☐ Sativa ☐ Indica ☐ Hybrid ☐ Not sure

Medium of Consumption: ☐ Flower ☐ Edible ☐ Concentrate ☐ Other _____

Method: ☐ Smoke ☐ Vape ☐ Ingest ☐ Other _____

Potency:
(Circle one)   🍁 1   🍁 2   🍁 3   🍁 4   🍁 5   🍁 6   🍁 7   🍁 8   🍁 9   🍁 10

THC % _____ CBD % _____ CBN % _____ Other % _____

Appearance and Taste

Aroma: _____

Color: _____

Flavor Notes: _____

Positive Effects:

☐ Creative ☐ Happy ☐ Energetic ☐ Euphoric ☐ Relaxed ☐ Talkative

☐ Uplifted ☐ Zen ☐ Other: _____

Negative Effects:

☐ Anxiety ☐ Cotton mouth ☐ Couch lock ☐ Dizziness ☐ Dry eyes

☐ Memory Problems ☐ Paranoid ☐ Other: _____

Helps with:

☐ General Pain ☐ Back Pain ☐ Anxiety ☐ Depression ☐ Concentration

☐ Sleep Problems ☐ Other: _____

Would try again?

☐ Yes ☐ No

Overall Rating:
(Circle one)   🍁 1   🍁 2   🍁 3   🍁 4   🍁 5   🍁 6   🍁 7   🍁 8   🍁 9   🍁 10

"Marijuana is a useful catalyst for specific optical and aural aesthetic perceptions. I apprehended the structure of certain pieces of jazz and classical music in a new manner under the influence of marijuana, and these apprehensions have remained valid in years of normal consciousness."
—Allen Ginsberg

Notes:

Strain Name: _____

Date: _____

Time taken: _____ Time it took to feel effects: _____

Strain Type: □ Sativa □ Indica □ Hybrid □ Not sure

Medium of Consumption: □ Flower □ Edible □ Concentrate □ Other _____

Method: □ Smoke □ Vape □ Ingest □ Other _____

Potency:
(Circle one)   🍁 1 🍁 2 🍁 3 🍁 4 🍁 5 🍁 6 🍁 7 🍁 8 🍁 9 🍁 10

THC % _____ CBD % _____ CBN % _____ Other % _____

Appearance and Taste

Aroma: _____

Color: _____

Flavor Notes: _____

Positive Effects:

□ Creative □ Happy □ Energetic □ Euphoric □ Relaxed □ Talkative

□ Uplifted □ Zen □ Other: _____

Negative Effects:

□ Anxiety □ Cotton mouth □ Couch lock □ Dizziness □ Dry eyes

□ Memory Problems □ Paranoid □ Other: _____

Helps with:

□ General Pain □ Back Pain □ Anxiety □ Depression □ Concentration

□ Sleep Problems □ Other: _____

Would try again?

□ Yes □ No

Overall Rating:
(Circle one)   🍁 1 🍁 2 🍁 3 🍁 4 🍁 5 🍁 6 🍁 7 🍁 8 🍁 9 🍁 10

Notes:

_____

_____

_____

_____

_____

_____

_____

_____

_____

_____

_____

_____

_____

_____

_____

_____

Tip: The last thing you want to do while high is to try and find a movie to watch or music to listen to. Make sure you have your media of choice queued up before you're too stoned to make a decision!

Strain Name: _____

Date: _____

Time taken: _____ Time it took to feel effects: _____

Strain Type: □ Sativa □ Indica □ Hybrid □ Not sure

Medium of Consumption: □ Flower □ Edible □ Concentrate □ Other _____

Method: □ Smoke □ Vape □ Ingest □ Other _____

Potency:
(Circle one) ❋ ❋ ❋ ❋ ❋ ❋ ❋ ❋ ❋ ❋
              1 2 3 4 5 6 7 8 9 10

THC % _____ CBD % _____ CBN % _____ Other % _____

Appearance and Taste

Aroma: _____

Color: _____

Flavor Notes: _____

Positive Effects:

□ **Creative** □ **Happy** □ **Energetic** □ **Euphoric** □ **Relaxed** □ **Talkative**

□ **Uplifted** □ **Zen** □ **Other:** _____

Negative Effects:

□ **Anxiety** □ **Cotton mouth** □ **Couch lock** □ **Dizziness** □ **Dry eyes**

□ **Memory Problems** □ **Paranoid** □ **Other:** _____

Helps with:

□ **General Pain** □ **Back Pain** □ **Anxiety** □ **Depression** □ **Concentration**

□ **Sleep Problems** □ **Other:** _____

Would try again?

□ **Yes** □ **No**

Overall Rating: ❋ ❋ ❋ ❋ ❋ ❋ ❋ ❋ ❋ ❋
(Circle one)   1 2 3 4 5 6 7 8 9 10

"Yes, I smoke shit, straight off the roach clip; I roach it for the blunted ones to approach it; Forward motion, make you sway like the ocean; The herb is more than just a powerful potion" —Cypress Hill, "I Want to Get High," *Black Sunday*

Notes:

Strain Name: _____

Date: _____

Time taken: _____ Time it took to feel effects: _____

Strain Type: □ Sativa   □ Indica   □ Hybrid   □ Not sure

Medium of Consumption: □ Flower   □ Edible   □ Concentrate   □ Other _____

Method: □ Smoke   □ Vape   □ Ingest   □ Other _____

Potency:
(Circle one)
1   2   3   4   5   6   7   8   9   10

THC % _____ CBD % _____ CBN % _____ Other % _____

Appearance and Taste

Aroma: _____

Color: _____

Flavor Notes: _____

Positive Effects:

□ Creative   □ Happy   □ Energetic   □ Euphoric   □ Relaxed   □ Talkative

□ Uplifted   □ Zen   □ Other: _____

Negative Effects:

□ Anxiety   □ Cotton mouth   □ Couch lock   □ Dizziness   □ Dry eyes

□ Memory Problems   □ Paranoid   □ Other: _____

Helps with:

□ General Pain   □ Back Pain   □ Anxiety   □ Depression   □ Concentration

□ Sleep Problems   □ Other: _____

Would try again?

□ Yes   □ No

Overall Rating:
(Circle one)
1   2   3   4   5   6   7   8   9   10

Tip: At some point in every stoner's life, they will want to smoke and not have a smoking device to do so. Grab an apple and remove the stem, in a matter of minutes you can have a homemade fruit pipe. Next, use a pencil to poke a hole through the side of the apple toward its core. Then make a hole going downwards from where you pulled the stem, this should be perpendicular to the first hole you made. Then just load your weed on the top of the apple where you removed the stem and light it."
(Andrew Salisbury, FatBuddhaGlass.com)

Notes:

_____

_____

_____

_____

_____

_____

_____

_____

_____

_____

_____

_____

_____

_____

_____

_____

Strain Name: _____

Date: _____

Time taken: _____ Time it took to feel effects: _____

Strain Type: □ Sativa   □ Indica   □ Hybrid   □ Not sure

Medium of Consumption: □ Flower   □ Edible   □ Concentrate   □ Other _____

Method: □ Smoke   □ Vape   □ Ingest   □ Other _____

Potency:
(Circle one)

1   2   3   4   5   6   7   8   9   10

THC % _____ CBD % _____ CBN % _____ Other % _____

Appearance and Taste

Aroma: _____

Color: _____

Flavor Notes: _____

Positive Effects:

□ **Creative**   □ **Happy**   □ **Energetic**   □ **Euphoric**   □ **Relaxed**   □ **Talkative**

□ **Uplifted**   □ **Zen**   □ **Other:** _____

Negative Effects:

□ **Anxiety**   □ **Cotton mouth**   □ **Couch lock**   □ **Dizziness**   □ **Dry eyes**

□ **Memory Problems**   □ **Paranoid**   □ **Other:** _____

Helps with:

□ **General Pain**   □ **Back Pain**   □ **Anxiety**   □ **Depression**   □ **Concentration**

□ **Sleep Problems**   □ **Other:** _____

Would try again?

□ **Yes**   □ **No**

Overall Rating:
(Circle one)

1   2   3   4   5   6   7   8   9   10

Notes:

"The illegality of cannabis is outrageous, an impediment to full utilization of a drug which helps produce the serenity and insight, sensitivity and fellowship so desperately needed in this increasingly mad and dangerous world."
—Carl Sagan

Strain Name: _____

Date: _____

Time taken: _____ Time it took to feel effects: _____

Strain Type: □ Sativa   □ Indica   □ Hybrid   □ Not sure

Medium of Consumption: □ Flower   □ Edible   □ Concentrate   □ Other _____

Method: □ Smoke   □ Vape   □ Ingest   □ Other _____

Potency:
(Circle one)
🌿 🌿 🌿 🌿 🌿 🌿 🌿 🌿 🌿 🌿
1   2   3   4   5   6   7   8   9   10

THC % _____ CBD % _____ CBN % _____ Other % _____

Appearance and Taste

Aroma: _____

Color: _____

Flavor Notes: _____

Positive Effects:

□ Creative   □ Happy   □ Energetic   □ Euphoric   □ Relaxed   □ Talkative

□ Uplifted   □ Zen   □ Other: _____

Negative Effects:

□ Anxiety   □ Cotton mouth   □ Couch lock   □ Dizziness   □ Dry eyes

□ Memory Problems   □ Paranoid   □ Other: _____

Helps with:

□ General Pain   □ Back Pain   □ Anxiety   □ Depression   □ Concentration

□ Sleep Problems   □ Other: _____

Would try again?

□ Yes   □ No

Overall Rating:
(Circle one)
🌿 🌿 🌿 🌿 🌿 🌿 🌿 🌿 🌿 🌿
1   2   3   4   5   6   7   8   9   10

Tip: Is your weed drying out? A great way to add moisture back into your bud is by adding a bit of orange peel to your container. This will add that sticky back to your icky!

Notes:

_____

_____

_____

_____

_____

_____

_____

_____

_____

_____

_____

_____

_____

_____

Strain Name: _____

Date: _____

Time taken: _____ Time it took to feel effects: _____

Strain Type: □ Sativa □ Indica □ Hybrid □ Not sure

Medium of Consumption: □ Flower □ Edible □ Concentrate □ Other _____

Method: □ Smoke □ Vape □ Ingest □ Other _____

Potency:
(Circle one)

🍁 1 🍁 2 🍁 3 🍁 4 🍁 5 🍁 6 🍁 7 🍁 8 🍁 9 🍁 10

THC % _____ CBD % _____ CBN % _____ Other % _____

Appearance and Taste

Aroma: _____

Color: _____

Flavor Notes: _____

Positive Effects:

□ Creative □ Happy □ Energetic □ Euphoric □ Relaxed □ Talkative

□ Uplifted □ Zen □ Other: _____

Negative Effects:

□ Anxiety □ Cotton mouth □ Couch lock □ Dizziness □ Dry eyes

□ Memory Problems □ Paranoid □ Other: _____

Helps with:

□ General Pain □ Back Pain □ Anxiety □ Depression □ Concentration

□ Sleep Problems □ Other: _____

Would try again?

□ Yes □ No

Overall Rating:
(Circle one)

🍁 1 🍁 2 🍁 3 🍁 4 🍁 5 🍁 6 🍁 7 🍁 8 🍁 9 🍁 10

> "More people get stoned in the Old Testament than in my jacuzzi." —Bill Maher

Notes:

_____

_____

_____

_____

_____

_____

_____

_____

_____

_____

_____

_____

_____

_____

_____

_____

_____

_____

_____

Strain Name: _____

Date: _____

Time taken: _____ Time it took to feel effects: _____

Strain Type: ☐ Sativa   ☐ Indica   ☐ Hybrid   ☐ Not sure

Medium of Consumption: ☐ Flower   ☐ Edible   ☐ Concentrate   ☐ Other _____

Method: ☐ Smoke   ☐ Vape   ☐ Ingest   ☐ Other _____

Potency:
(Circle one)   1   2   3   4   5   6   7   8   9   10

THC % _____   CBD % _____   CBN % _____   Other % _____

Appearance and Taste

Aroma: _____

Color: _____

Flavor Notes: _____

Positive Effects:

☐ Creative   ☐ Happy   ☐ Energetic   ☐ Euphoric   ☐ Relaxed   ☐ Talkative

☐ Uplifted   ☐ Zen   ☐ Other: _____

Negative Effects:

☐ Anxiety   ☐ Cotton mouth   ☐ Couch lock   ☐ Dizziness   ☐ Dry eyes

☐ Memory Problems   ☐ Paranoid   ☐ Other: _____

Helps with:

☐ General Pain   ☐ Back Pain   ☐ Anxiety   ☐ Depression   ☐ Concentration

☐ Sleep Problems   ☐ Other: _____

Would try again?

☐ Yes   ☐ No

Overall Rating:
(Circle one)   1   2   3   4   5   6   7   8   9   10

Notes:

_____

_____

_____

_____

_____

_____

_____

_____

_____

_____

_____

_____

_____

_____

_____

_____

Tip: "Sour candy will get your saliva production going again, ending the uncomfortable dry mouth. Suck on candy while smoking to prevent it." (Alden, *World of Weed*)

Strain Name: _____

Date: _____

Time taken: _____   Time it took to feel effects: _____

Strain Type: □ Sativa   □ Indica   □ Hybrid   □ Not sure

Medium of Consumption: □ Flower   □ Edible   □ Concentrate   □ Other _____

Method: □ Smoke   □ Vape   □ Ingest   □ Other _____

Potency:
(Circle one)   🌿 1   🌿 2   🌿 3   🌿 4   🌿 5   🌿 6   🌿 7   🌿 8   🌿 9   🌿 10

THC % _____ CBD % _____ CBN % _____ Other % _____

Appearance and Taste

Aroma: _____

Color: _____

Flavor Notes: _____

Positive Effects:

□ Creative   □ Happy   □ Energetic   □ Euphoric   □ Relaxed   □ Talkative

□ Uplifted   □ Zen   □ Other: _____

Negative Effects:

□ Anxiety   □ Cotton mouth   □ Couch lock   □ Dizziness   □ Dry eyes

□ Memory Problems   □ Paranoid   □ Other: _____

Helps with:

□ General Pain   □ Back Pain   □ Anxiety   □ Depression   □ Concentration

□ Sleep Problems   □ Other: _____

Would try again?

□ Yes   □ No

Overall Rating:
(Circle one)   🌿 1   🌿 2   🌿 3   🌿 4   🌿 5   🌿 6   🌿 7   🌿 8   🌿 9   🌿 10

There is absolutely nothing wrong with the responsible use of marijuana by adults and it should be of no interest or concern to the government. They have no business knowing whethere we smoke or why we smoke." —Keith Stroup

Notes:

Strain Name: _____

Date: _____

Time taken: _____ Time it took to feel effects: _____

Strain Type: ☐ Sativa ☐ Indica ☐ Hybrid ☐ Not sure

Medium of Consumption: ☐ Flower ☐ Edible ☐ Concentrate ☐ Other _____

Method: ☐ Smoke ☐ Vape ☐ Ingest ☐ Other _____

Potency:
(Circle one)
🍁 🍁 🍁 🍁 🍁 🍁 🍁 🍁 🍁 🍁
1　　2　　3　　4　　5　　6　　7　　8　　9　　10

THC % _____ CBD % _____ CBN % _____ Other % _____

Appearance and Taste

Aroma: _____

Color: _____

Flavor Notes: _____

Positive Effects:

☐ **Creative** ☐ **Happy** ☐ **Energetic** ☐ **Euphoric** ☐ **Relaxed** ☐ **Talkative**

☐ **Uplifted** ☐ **Zen** ☐ **Other:** _____

Negative Effects:

☐ **Anxiety** ☐ **Cotton mouth** ☐ **Couch lock** ☐ **Dizziness** ☐ **Dry eyes**

☐ **Memory Problems** ☐ **Paranoid** ☐ **Other:** _____

Helps with:

☐ **General Pain** ☐ **Back Pain** ☐ **Anxiety** ☐ **Depression** ☐ **Concentration**

☐ **Sleep Problems** ☐ **Other:** _____

Would try again?

☐ **Yes** ☐ **No**

Overall Rating:
(Circle one)
🍁 🍁 🍁 🍁 🍁 🍁 🍁 🍁 🍁 🍁
1　　2　　3　　4　　5　　6　　7　　8　　9　　10

Tip: Have a dedicated pipe cleaner in your arsenal to clear out any potential clogs (especially when you want to burn and don't have the time for a full cleaning).

Notes:

Strain Name: _____

Date: _____

Time taken: _____ Time it took to feel effects: _____

Strain Type: □ Sativa □ Indica □ Hybrid □ Not sure

Medium of Consumption: □ Flower □ Edible □ Concentrate □ Other _____

Method: □ Smoke □ Vape □ Ingest □ Other _____

Potency:
(Circle one) 🍁 🍁 🍁 🍁 🍁 🍁 🍁 🍁 🍁 🍁
        1   2   3   4   5   6   7   8   9   10

THC % _____ CBD % _____ CBN % _____ Other % _____

Appearance and Taste

Aroma: _____

Color: _____

Flavor Notes: _____

Positive Effects:

□ Creative □ Happy □ Energetic □ Euphoric □ Relaxed □ Talkative

□ Uplifted □ Zen □ Other: _____

Negative Effects:

□ Anxiety □ Cotton mouth □ Couch lock □ Dizziness □ Dry eyes

□ Memory Problems □ Paranoid □ Other: _____

Helps with:

□ General Pain □ Back Pain □ Anxiety □ Depression □ Concentration

□ Sleep Problems □ Other: _____

Would try again?

□ Yes □ No

Overall Rating: 🍁 🍁 🍁 🍁 🍁 🍁 🍁 🍁 🍁 🍁
(Circle one)   1   2   3   4   5   6   7   8   9   10

Notes:

_____

_____

_____

_____

_____

_____

_____

_____

_____

_____

_____

_____

_____

_____

_____

"Today, I believe there is no such thing as the recreational use of cannabis. The concept is equally embraced by prohibitionists and self-professed stoners, but it is self-limiting and profoundly unhealthy. Defining cannabis consumption as elective recreation ignores fundamental human biology and history, and devalues the very real benefits the plant provides. . . ." —**Steve DeAngelo,** _The Cannabis Manifesto: A New Paradigm for Wellness_

Strain Name: _____

Date: _____

Time taken: _____ Time it took to feel effects: _____

Strain Type: ☐ Sativa ☐ Indica ☐ Hybrid ☐ Not sure

Medium of Consumption: ☐ Flower ☐ Edible ☐ Concentrate ☐ Other _____

Method: ☐ Smoke ☐ Vape ☐ Ingest ☐ Other _____

Potency:
(Circle one)

🍁 🍁 🍁 🍁 🍁 🍁 🍁 🍁 🍁 🍁
1   2   3   4   5   6   7   8   9   10

THC % _____ CBD % _____ CBN % _____ Other % _____

Appearance and Taste

Aroma: _____

Color: _____

Flavor Notes: _____

Positive Effects:

☐ Creative ☐ Happy ☐ Energetic ☐ Euphoric ☐ Relaxed ☐ Talkative

☐ Uplifted ☐ Zen ☐ Other: _____

Negative Effects:

☐ Anxiety ☐ Cotton mouth ☐ Couch lock ☐ Dizziness ☐ Dry eyes

☐ Memory Problems ☐ Paranoid ☐ Other: _____

Helps with:

☐ General Pain ☐ Back Pain ☐ Anxiety ☐ Depression ☐ Concentration

☐ Sleep Problems ☐ Other: _____

Would try again?

☐ Yes ☐ No

Overall Rating:
(Circle one)

🍁 🍁 🍁 🍁 🍁 🍁 🍁 🍁 🍁 🍁
1   2   3   4   5   6   7   8   9   10

Tip: "A helpful and possibly overlooked weed life hack for stoners is the way you hold your lighter when lighting a joint. The flame on a lighter will always remain vertical so matter which way you turn it. Rather than tilting your head forward when lighting your joint, tilt your head back and the heat will rise away from your face, therefore reducing the chances of cinged eyelashes and eyebrows." (Hydro Wilson, *Potent*)

Notes:

Strain Name: _____

Date: _____

Time taken: _____ Time it took to feel effects: _____

Strain Type: □ Sativa □ Indica □ Hybrid □ Not sure

Medium of Consumption: □ Flower □ Edible □ Concentrate □ Other _____

Method: □ Smoke □ Vape □ Ingest □ Other _____

Potency:
(Circle one)
1 2 3 4 5 6 7 8 9 10

THC % _____ CBD % _____ CBN % _____ Other % _____

Appearance and Taste

Aroma: _____

Color: _____

Flavor Notes: _____

Positive Effects:

□ **Creative** □ **Happy** □ **Energetic** □ **Euphoric** □ **Relaxed** □ **Talkative**

□ **Uplifted** □ **Zen** □ **Other:** _____

Negative Effects:

□ **Anxiety** □ **Cotton mouth** □ **Couch lock** □ **Dizziness** □ **Dry eyes**

□ **Memory Problems** □ **Paranoid** □ **Other:** _____

Helps with:

□ **General Pain** □ **Back Pain** □ **Anxiety** □ **Depression** □ **Concentration**

□ **Sleep Problems** □ **Other:** _____

Would try again?

□ Yes □ No

Overall Rating:
(Circle one)
1 2 3 4 5 6 7 8 9 10

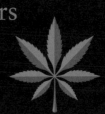

"I've been smoking marijuana for forty-four years now and . . . I think it's a tremendous blessing."
—Lester Grinspoon

Notes:

Strain Name: _____

Date: _____

Time taken: _____ Time it took to feel effects: _____

Strain Type: □ Sativa   □ Indica   □ Hybrid   □ Not sure

Medium of Consumption: □ Flower   □ Edible   □ Concentrate   □ Other _____

Method: □ Smoke   □ Vape   □ Ingest   □ Other _____

Potency:
(Circle one)
1   2   3   4   5   6   7   8   9   10

THC % _____ CBD % _____ CBN % _____ Other % _____

Appearance and Taste

Aroma: _____

Color: _____

Flavor Notes: _____

Positive Effects:

□ **Creative**   □ **Happy**   □ **Energetic**   □ **Euphoric**   □ **Relaxed**   □ **Talkative**

□ **Uplifted**   □ **Zen**   □ **Other:** _____

Negative Effects:

□ **Anxiety**   □ **Cotton mouth**   □ **Couch lock**   □ **Dizziness**   □ **Dry eyes**

□ **Memory Problems**   □ **Paranoid**   □ **Other:** _____

Helps with:

□ **General Pain**   □ **Back Pain**   □ **Anxiety**   □ **Depression**   □ **Concentration**

□ **Sleep Problems**   □ **Other:** _____

Would try again?

□ Yes   □ No

Overall Rating:
(Circle one)
1   2   3   4   5   6   7   8   9   10

Notes:

_____

_____

_____

_____

_____

_____

_____

_____

_____

_____

_____

_____

_____

_____

_____

Tip: "Mason jars are great for storage. Use a humidipack and you are set for life with fresh, tasty weed. 62% is a good number." (Morgan, 420GreenThumb.com)

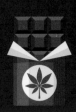

Strain Name: _____

Date: _____

Time taken: _____   Time it took to feel effects: _____

Strain Type: □ Sativa   □ Indica   □ Hybrid   □ Not sure

Medium of Consumption: □ Flower   □ Edible   □ Concentrate   □ Other _____

Method: □ Smoke   □ Vape   □ Ingest   □ Other _____

Potency:
(Circle one)   ✳ 1   ✳ 2   ✳ 3   ✳ 4   ✳ 5   ✳ 6   ✳ 7   ✳ 8   ✳ 9   ✳ 10

THC % _____   CBD % _____   CBN % _____   Other % _____

Appearance and Taste

Aroma: _____

Color: _____

Flavor Notes: _____

Positive Effects:

□ Creative   □ Happy   □ Energetic   □ Euphoric   □ Relaxed   □ Talkative

□ Uplifted   □ Zen   □ Other: _____

Negative Effects:

□ Anxiety   □ Cotton mouth   □ Couch lock   □ Dizziness   □ Dry eyes

□ Memory Problems   □ Paranoid   □ Other: _____

Helps with:

□ General Pain   □ Back Pain   □ Anxiety   □ Depression   □ Concentration

□ Sleep Problems   □ Other: _____

Would try again?

□ Yes   □ No

Overall Rating:
(Circle one)   ✳ 1   ✳ 2   ✳ 3   ✳ 4   ✳ 5   ✳ 6   ✳ 7   ✳ 8   ✳ 9   ✳ 10

> "Stop killing each other, man.
> Let's just smoke a blunt."
> —Tupac Shakur

Notes:

_____

_____

_____

_____

_____

_____

_____

_____

_____

_____

_____

_____

_____

_____

_____

_____

_____

Strain Name: _____

Date: _____

Time taken: _____ Time it took to feel effects: _____

Strain Type: □ Sativa □ Indica □ Hybrid □ Not sure

Medium of Consumption: □ Flower □ Edible □ Concentrate □ Other _____

Method: □ Smoke □ Vape □ Ingest □ Other _____

Potency:
(Circle one)

1 2 3 4 5 6 7 8 9 10

THC % _____ CBD % _____ CBN % _____ Other % _____

Appearance and Taste

Aroma: _____

Color: _____

Flavor Notes: _____

Positive Effects:

□ Creative □ Happy □ Energetic □ Euphoric □ Relaxed □ Talkative

□ Uplifted □ Zen □ Other: _____

Negative Effects:

□ Anxiety □ Cotton mouth □ Couch lock □ Dizziness □ Dry eyes

□ Memory Problems □ Paranoid □ Other: _____

Helps with:

□ General Pain □ Back Pain □ Anxiety □ Depression □ Concentration

□ Sleep Problems □ Other: _____

Would try again?

□ Yes □ No

Overall Rating:
(Circle one)

1 2 3 4 5 6 7 8 9 10

Tip: "Any flying disc or Frisbee with a concave edge is very helpful when rolling blunts and joints: the cupped outline keeps loose weed from falling onto the floor." (Daniel Jones, *The Cannabist*)

Notes:

Strain Name: _____

Date: _____

Time taken: _____ Time it took to feel effects: _____

Strain Type: □ Sativa   □ Indica   □ Hybrid   □ Not sure

Medium of Consumption: □ Flower   □ Edible   □ Concentrate   □ Other _____

Method: □ Smoke   □ Vape   □ Ingest   □ Other _____

Potency:
(Circle one)
🌿 🌿 🌿 🌿 🌿 🌿 🌿 🌿 🌿 🌿
1   2   3   4   5   6   7   8   9   10

THC % _____ CBD % _____ CBN % _____ Other % _____

Appearance and Taste

Aroma: _____

Color: _____

Flavor Notes: _____

Positive Effects:

□ **Creative**   □ **Happy**   □ **Energetic**   □ **Euphoric**   □ **Relaxed**   □ **Talkative**

□ **Uplifted**   □ **Zen**   □ **Other:** _____

Negative Effects:

□ **Anxiety**   □ **Cotton mouth**   □ **Couch lock**   □ **Dizziness**   □ **Dry eyes**

□ **Memory Problems**   □ **Paranoid**   □ **Other:** _____

Helps with:

□ **General Pain**   □ **Back Pain**   □ **Anxiety**   □ **Depression**   □ **Concentration**

□ **Sleep Problems**   □ **Other:** _____

Would try again?

□ Yes   □ No

Overall Rating:
(Circle one)
🌿 🌿 🌿 🌿 🌿 🌿 🌿 🌿 🌿 🌿
1   2   3   4   5   6   7   8   9   10

Notes:

_____

_____

_____

_____

_____

_____

_____

_____

_____

_____

_____

_____

_____

_____

_____

"It makes me feel the way I need to feel."
—Snoop Dogg

Strain Name: _____

Date: _____

Time taken: _____ Time it took to feel effects: _____

Strain Type: □ Sativa   □ Indica   □ Hybrid   □ Not sure

Medium of Consumption: □ Flower   □ Edible   □ Concentrate   □ Other _____

Method: □ Smoke   □ Vape   □ Ingest   □ Other _____

Potency:
(Circle one)
1   2   3   4   5   6   7   8   9   10

THC % _____ CBD % _____ CBN % _____ Other % _____

Appearance and Taste

Aroma: _____

Color: _____

Flavor Notes: _____

Positive Effects:

□ Creative   □ Happy   □ Energetic   □ Euphoric   □ Relaxed   □ Talkative

□ Uplifted   □ Zen   □ Other: _____

Negative Effects:

□ Anxiety   □ Cotton mouth   □ Couch lock   □ Dizziness   □ Dry eyes

□ Memory Problems   □ Paranoid   □ Other: _____

Helps with:

□ General Pain   □ Back Pain   □ Anxiety   □ Depression   □ Concentration

□ Sleep Problems   □ Other: _____

Would try again?

□ Yes   □ No

Overall Rating:
(Circle one)
1   2   3   4   5   6   7   8   9   10

Tip: Have your weed in a clear jar? One way to keep it fresh is to "wrap black construction paper around your weed jar to prevent exposure to light, keeping your bud fresher for longer." (Tanya Chen, *Buzzfeed*)

Notes:

Strain Name: _____

Date: _____

Time taken: _____   Time it took to feel effects: _____

Strain Type: □ Sativa   □ Indica   □ Hybrid   □ Not sure

Medium of Consumption: □ Flower   □ Edible   □ Concentrate   □ Other _____

Method: □ Smoke   □ Vape   □ Ingest   □ Other _____

Potency:
(Circle one)   🍁 1   🍁 2   🍁 3   🍁 4   🍁 5   🍁 6   🍁 7   🍁 8   🍁 9   🍁 10

THC % _____ CBD % _____ CBN % _____ Other % _____

Appearance and Taste

Aroma: _____

Color: _____

Flavor Notes: _____

Positive Effects:

□ Creative   □ Happy   □ Energetic   □ Euphoric   □ Relaxed   □ Talkative

□ Uplifted   □ Zen   □ Other: _____

Negative Effects:

□ Anxiety   □ Cotton mouth   □ Couch lock   □ Dizziness   □ Dry eyes

□ Memory Problems   □ Paranoid   □ Other: _____

Helps with:

□ General Pain   □ Back Pain   □ Anxiety   □ Depression   □ Concentration

□ Sleep Problems   □ Other: _____

Would try again?

□ Yes   □ No

Overall Rating:
(Circle one)   🍁 1   🍁 2   🍁 3   🍁 4   🍁 5   🍁 6   🍁 7   🍁 8   🍁 9   🍁 10

"Few things nicer than getting baked, walking around New York on a sunny day and eavesdropping on couples who are arguing." —Seth Rogen

Notes:

Strain Name: _____

Date: _____

Time taken: _____ Time it took to feel effects: _____

Strain Type: ☐ Sativa ☐ Indica ☐ Hybrid ☐ Not sure

Medium of Consumption: ☐ Flower ☐ Edible ☐ Concentrate ☐ Other _____

Method: ☐ Smoke ☐ Vape ☐ Ingest ☐ Other _____

Potency:
(Circle one)

🍁 1 🍁 2 🍁 3 🍁 4 🍁 5 🍁 6 🍁 7 🍁 8 🍁 9 🍁 10

THC % _____ CBD % _____ CBN % _____ Other % _____

Appearance and Taste

Aroma: _____

Color: _____

Flavor Notes: _____

Positive Effects:

☐ Creative ☐ Happy ☐ Energetic ☐ Euphoric ☐ Relaxed ☐ Talkative

☐ Uplifted ☐ Zen ☐ Other: _____

Negative Effects:

☐ Anxiety ☐ Cotton mouth ☐ Couch lock ☐ Dizziness ☐ Dry eyes

☐ Memory Problems ☐ Paranoid ☐ Other: _____

Helps with:

☐ General Pain ☐ Back Pain ☐ Anxiety ☐ Depression ☐ Concentration

☐ Sleep Problems ☐ Other: _____

Would try again?

☐ Yes ☐ No

Overall Rating:
(Circle one)

🍁 1 🍁 2 🍁 3 🍁 4 🍁 5 🍁 6 🍁 7 🍁 8 🍁 9 🍁 10

Notes:

_____

_____

_____

_____

_____

_____

_____

_____

_____

_____

_____

_____

_____

_____

_____

_____

Tip: Many grinders have a keef catcher, and while we are all saving it for a rainy day, don't let it sit forever. While it'll most likely stay usable for an extended period of time, it can oftentimes lose its potency. A good test is to give it a smell. If it's stinky, it's good. If it has no smell, it's most likely lost its potency.

Strain Name: _____

Date: _____

Time taken: _____ Time it took to feel effects: _____

Strain Type: □ Sativa □ Indica □ Hybrid □ Not sure

Medium of Consumption: □ Flower □ Edible □ Concentrate □ Other _____

Method: □ Smoke □ Vape □ Ingest □ Other _____

Potency:
(Circle one)

      1   2   3   4   5   6   7   8   9   10

THC % _____ CBD % _____ CBN % _____ Other % _____

Appearance and Taste

Aroma: _____

Color: _____

Flavor Notes: _____

Positive Effects:

□ **Creative** □ **Happy** □ **Energetic** □ **Euphoric** □ **Relaxed** □ **Talkative**

□ **Uplifted** □ **Zen** □ **Other:** _____

Negative Effects:

□ **Anxiety** □ **Cotton mouth** □ **Couch lock** □ **Dizziness** □ **Dry eyes**

□ **Memory Problems** □ **Paranoid** □ **Other:** _____

Helps with:

□ **General Pain** □ **Back Pain** □ **Anxiety** □ **Depression** □ **Concentration**

□ **Sleep Problems** □ **Other:** _____

Would try again?

□ **Yes** □ **No**

Overall Rating:
(Circle one)

      1   2   3   4   5   6   7   8   9   10

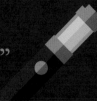

"A friend with weed is a friend indeed . . ."
—Pops O'Donnell

Notes:

Strain Name: _____

Date: _____

Time taken: _____ Time it took to feel effects: _____

Strain Type: □ Sativa   □ Indica   □ Hybrid   □ Not sure

Medium of Consumption: □ Flower   □ Edible   □ Concentrate   □ Other _____

Method: □ Smoke   □ Vape   □ Ingest   □ Other _____

Potency:
(Circle one)
🍁 1 🍁 2 🍁 3 🍁 4 🍁 5 🍁 6 🍁 7 🍁 8 🍁 9 🍁 10

THC % _____ CBD % _____ CBN % _____ Other % _____

Appearance and Taste

Aroma: _____

Color: _____

Flavor Notes: _____

Positive Effects:

□ Creative   □ Happy   □ Energetic   □ Euphoric   □ Relaxed   □ Talkative

□ Uplifted   □ Zen   □ Other: _____

Negative Effects:

□ Anxiety   □ Cotton mouth   □ Couch lock   □ Dizziness   □ Dry eyes

□ Memory Problems   □ Paranoid   □ Other: _____

Helps with:

□ General Pain   □ Back Pain   □ Anxiety   □ Depression   □ Concentration

□ Sleep Problems   □ Other: _____

Would try again?

□ Yes   □ No

Overall Rating:
(Circle one)
🍁 1 🍁 2 🍁 3 🍁 4 🍁 5 🍁 6 🍁 7 🍁 8 🍁 9 🍁 10

Tip: For those MacGyver stoners who love to create their own smoking vessels, make sure to stay away from any metals that would be harmful to your lungs. That means the easily made Coca Cola can bowls!

Notes:

_____

_____

_____

_____

_____

_____

_____

_____

_____

_____

_____

_____

_____

_____

_____

_____

_____

Strain Name: _____

Date: _____

Time taken: _____ Time it took to feel effects: _____

Strain Type: □ Sativa □ Indica □ Hybrid □ Not sure

Medium of Consumption: □ Flower □ Edible □ Concentrate □ Other _____

Method: □ Smoke □ Vape □ Ingest □ Other _____

Potency:
(Circle one)
   1   2   3   4   5   6   7   8   9   10

THC % _____ CBD % _____ CBN % _____ Other % _____

Appearance and Taste

Aroma: _____

Color: _____

Flavor Notes: _____

Positive Effects:

□ Creative □ Happy □ Energetic □ Euphoric □ Relaxed □ Talkative

□ Uplifted □ Zen □ Other: _____

Negative Effects:

□ Anxiety □ Cotton mouth □ Couch lock □ Dizziness □ Dry eyes

□ Memory Problems □ Paranoid □ Other: _____

Helps with:

□ General Pain □ Back Pain □ Anxiety □ Depression □ Concentration

□ Sleep Problems □ Other: _____

Would try again?

□ Yes □ No

Overall Rating:
(Circle one)
   1   2   3   4   5   6   7   8   9   10

Notes:

_____

_____

_____

_____

_____

_____

_____

_____

_____

_____

_____

_____

_____

_____

_____

_____

"Dope will get you through times of no money better than money will get you through times of no dope."
—Freewheelin' Franklin

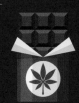

Strain Name: _____

Date: _____

Time taken: _____ Time it took to feel effects: _____

Strain Type: □ Sativa □ Indica □ Hybrid □ Not sure

Medium of Consumption: □ Flower □ Edible □ Concentrate □ Other _____

Method: □ Smoke □ Vape □ Ingest □ Other _____

Potency:
(Circle one)
1 2 3 4 5 6 7 8 9 10

THC % _____ CBD % _____ CBN % _____ Other % _____

Appearance and Taste

Aroma: _____

Color: _____

Flavor Notes: _____

Positive Effects:

□ Creative □ Happy □ Energetic □ Euphoric □ Relaxed □ Talkative

□ Uplifted □ Zen □ Other: _____

Negative Effects:

□ Anxiety □ Cotton mouth □ Couch lock □ Dizziness □ Dry eyes

□ Memory Problems □ Paranoid □ Other: _____

Helps with:

□ General Pain □ Back Pain □ Anxiety □ Depression □ Concentration

□ Sleep Problems □ Other: _____

Would try again?

□ Yes □ No

Overall Rating:
(Circle one)
1 2 3 4 5 6 7 8 9 10

Tip: Don't have a grinder on hand? "Grab a penny and clean it thoroughly, then put your marijuana in a pill box, drop the penny inside, close it up, and shake. Keep on shaking. After a vigorous workout you'll be left with a some evenly cut marijuana." (Maria Loreto, The Frest Toast)

Notes:

Strain Name: _____

Date: _____

Time taken: _____ Time it took to feel effects: _____

Strain Type: □ Sativa □ Indica □ Hybrid □ Not sure

Medium of Consumption: □ Flower □ Edible □ Concentrate □ Other _____

Method: □ Smoke □ Vape □ Ingest □ Other _____

Potency:
(Circle one) 🍁 🍁 🍁 🍁 🍁 🍁 🍁 🍁 🍁 🍁
              1   2   3   4   5   6   7   8   9   10

THC % _____ CBD % _____ CBN % _____ Other % _____

Appearance and Taste

Aroma: _____

Color: _____

Flavor Notes: _____

Positive Effects:

□ Creative   □ Happy   □ Energetic   □ Euphoric   □ Relaxed   □ Talkative

□ Uplifted   □ Zen   □ Other: _____

Negative Effects:

□ Anxiety   □ Cotton mouth   □ Couch lock   □ Dizziness   □ Dry eyes

□ Memory Problems   □ Paranoid   □ Other: _____

Helps with:

□ General Pain   □ Back Pain   □ Anxiety   □ Depression   □ Concentration

□ Sleep Problems   □ Other: _____

Would try again?

□ Yes   □ No

Overall Rating:
(Circle one) 🍁 🍁 🍁 🍁 🍁 🍁 🍁 🍁 🍁 🍁
              1   2   3   4   5   6   7   8   9   10

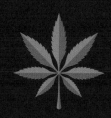
Notes:

Strain Name: _____

Date: _____

Time taken: _____ Time it took to feel effects: _____

Strain Type: ☐ Sativa   ☐ Indica   ☐ Hybrid   ☐ Not sure

Medium of Consumption: ☐ Flower   ☐ Edible   ☐ Concentrate   ☐ Other _____

Method: ☐ Smoke   ☐ Vape   ☐ Ingest   ☐ Other _____

Potency:
(Circle one)
1   2   3   4   5   6   7   8   9   10

THC % _____ CBD % _____ CBN % _____ Other % _____

Appearance and Taste

Aroma: _____

Color: _____

Flavor Notes: _____

Positive Effects:

☐ Creative   ☐ Happy   ☐ Energetic   ☐ Euphoric   ☐ Relaxed   ☐ Talkative

☐ Uplifted   ☐ Zen   ☐ Other: _____

Negative Effects:

☐ Anxiety   ☐ Cotton mouth   ☐ Couch lock   ☐ Dizziness   ☐ Dry eyes

☐ Memory Problems   ☐ Paranoid   ☐ Other: _____

Helps with:

☐ General Pain   ☐ Back Pain   ☐ Anxiety   ☐ Depression   ☐ Concentration

☐ Sleep Problems   ☐ Other: _____

Would try again?

☐ Yes   ☐ No

Overall Rating:
(Circle one)
1   2   3   4   5   6   7   8   9   10

Notes:

_____

_____

_____

_____

_____

_____

_____

_____

_____

_____

_____

_____

_____

_____

_____

_____

_____

Tip: "Don't cry over spilled milk, or weed. You can use nylon (or a sock—preferably a clean one) to wrap around the vacuum suction. Turn on your vacuum and start sucking up that green, then when you're finished and the vacuum is turned off—your weed is cleaned up and you can still use it!" (Everything 420)

Strain Name: _____

Date: _____

Time taken: _____ Time it took to feel effects: _____

Strain Type: □ Sativa   □ Indica   □ Hybrid   □ Not sure

Medium of Consumption: □ Flower   □ Edible   □ Concentrate   □ Other _____

Method: □ Smoke   □ Vape   □ Ingest   □ Other _____

Potency:
(Circle one)   🍁 1   🍁 2   🍁 3   🍁 4   🍁 5   🍁 6   🍁 7   🍁 8   🍁 9   🍁 10

THC % _____ CBD % _____ CBN % _____ Other % _____

Appearance and Taste

Aroma: _____

Color: _____

Flavor Notes: _____

Positive Effects:

□ **Creative**   □ **Happy**   □ **Energetic**   □ **Euphoric**   □ **Relaxed**   □ **Talkative**

□ **Uplifted**   □ **Zen**   □ **Other:** _____

Negative Effects:

□ **Anxiety**   □ **Cotton mouth**   □ **Couch lock**   □ **Dizziness**   □ **Dry eyes**

□ **Memory Problems**   □ **Paranoid**   □ **Other:** _____

Helps with:

□ **General Pain**   □ **Back Pain**   □ **Anxiety**   □ **Depression**   □ **Concentration**

□ **Sleep Problems**   □ **Other:** _____

Would try again?

□ **Yes**   □ **No**

Overall Rating: 🍁 1   🍁 2   🍁 3   🍁 4   🍁 5   🍁 6   🍁 7   🍁 8   🍁 9   🍁 10
(Circle one)

"We don't have time for questions. We need marijuana now, as much of it as possible! Like a big bag of it." —Kumar Patel, *Harold & Kumar Go to White Castle*

Notes:

Strain Name: _____

Date: _____

Time taken: _____   Time it took to feel effects: _____

Strain Type: □ Sativa   □ Indica   □ Hybrid   □ Not sure

Medium of Consumption: □ Flower   □ Edible   □ Concentrate   □ Other _____

Method: □ Smoke   □ Vape   □ Ingest   □ Other _____

Potency:
(Circle one)
1   2   3   4   5   6   7   8   9   10

THC % _____ CBD % _____ CBN % _____ Other % _____

Appearance and Taste

Aroma: _____

Color: _____

Flavor Notes: _____

Positive Effects:

□ Creative   □ Happy   □ Energetic   □ Euphoric   □ Relaxed   □ Talkative

□ Uplifted   □ Zen   □ Other: _____

Negative Effects:

□ Anxiety   □ Cotton mouth   □ Couch lock   □ Dizziness   □ Dry eyes

□ Memory Problems   □ Paranoid   □ Other: _____

Helps with:

□ General Pain   □ Back Pain   □ Anxiety   □ Depression   □ Concentration

□ Sleep Problems   □ Other: _____

Would try again?

□ Yes   □ No

Overall Rating:
(Circle one)
1   2   3   4   5   6   7   8   9   10

Tip: For those that need to be discreet and are relegated to smoking in the bathroom, in addition to keeping the fan on, place a damp towel directly under the door.

Notes:

Strain Name: _____

Date: _____

Time taken: _____ Time it took to feel effects: _____

Strain Type: □ Sativa □ Indica □ Hybrid □ Not sure

Medium of Consumption: □ Flower □ Edible □ Concentrate □ Other _____

Method: □ Smoke □ Vape □ Ingest □ Other _____

Potency:
(Circle one) 🌿 🌿 🌿 🌿 🌿 🌿 🌿 🌿 🌿 🌿
            1   2   3   4   5   6   7   8   9   10

THC % _____ CBD % _____ CBN % _____ Other % _____

Appearance and Taste

Aroma: _____

Color: _____

Flavor Notes: _____

Positive Effects:

□ Creative □ Happy □ Energetic □ Euphoric □ Relaxed □ Talkative

□ Uplifted □ Zen □ Other: _____

Negative Effects:

□ Anxiety □ Cotton mouth □ Couch lock □ Dizziness □ Dry eyes

□ Memory Problems □ Paranoid □ Other: _____

Helps with:

□ General Pain □ Back Pain □ Anxiety □ Depression □ Concentration

□ Sleep Problems □ Other: _____

Would try again?

□ Yes □ No

Overall Rating:
(Circle one) 🌿 🌿 🌿 🌿 🌿 🌿 🌿 🌿 🌿 🌿
            1   2   3   4   5   6   7   8   9   10

Notes:

_____

_____

_____

_____

_____

_____

_____

_____

_____

_____

_____

_____

_____

_____

_____

_____

"Let us burn one from end to end, and pass it over to me my friend." –Ben Harper, "Burn One Down," *Fight for Your Mind*

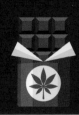

Strain Name: _____

Date: _____

Time taken: _____ Time it took to feel effects: _____

Strain Type: □ Sativa □ Indica □ Hybrid □ Not sure

Medium of Consumption: □ Flower □ Edible □ Concentrate □ Other _____

Method: □ Smoke □ Vape □ Ingest □ Other _____

Potency:
(Circle one)   1   2   3   4   5   6   7   8   9   10

THC % _____ CBD % _____ CBN % _____ Other % _____

Appearance and Taste

Aroma: _____

Color: _____

Flavor Notes: _____

Positive Effects:

□ Creative   □ Happy   □ Energetic   □ Euphoric   □ Relaxed   □ Talkative

□ Uplifted   □ Zen   □ Other: _____

Negative Effects:

□ Anxiety   □ Cotton mouth   □ Couch lock   □ Dizziness   □ Dry eyes

□ Memory Problems   □ Paranoid   □ Other: _____

Helps with:

□ General Pain   □ Back Pain   □ Anxiety   □ Depression   □ Concentration

□ Sleep Problems   □ Other: _____

Would try again?

□ Yes   □ No

Overall Rating:
(Circle one)   1   2   3   4   5   6   7   8   9   10

Tip: "Adding lemon juice to your bong water will reduce the buildup of resin on the glass. The acidity of the lemon juice is what helps break down resin and will act as an active cleaning agent while smoking." (StonerDays.com)

Notes:

Strain Name: _____

Date: _____

Time taken: _____   Time it took to feel effects: _____

Strain Type: □ Sativa   □ Indica   □ Hybrid   □ Not sure

Medium of Consumption: □ Flower   □ Edible   □ Concentrate   □ Other _____

Method: □ Smoke   □ Vape   □ Ingest   □ Other _____

Potency:
(Circle one)   🍁 1   🍁 2   🍁 3   🍁 4   🍁 5   🍁 6   🍁 7   🍁 8   🍁 9   🍁 10

THC % _____   CBD % _____   CBN % _____   Other % _____

Appearance and Taste

Aroma: _____

Color: _____

Flavor Notes: _____

Positive Effects:

□ Creative   □ Happy   □ Energetic   □ Euphoric   □ Relaxed   □ Talkative

□ Uplifted   □ Zen   □ Other: _____

Negative Effects:

□ Anxiety   □ Cotton mouth   □ Couch lock   □ Dizziness   □ Dry eyes

□ Memory Problems   □ Paranoid   □ Other: _____

Helps with:

□ General Pain   □ Back Pain   □ Anxiety   □ Depression   □ Concentration

□ Sleep Problems   □ Other: _____

Would try again?

□ Yes   □ No

Overall Rating:
(Circle one)   🍁 1   🍁 2   🍁 3   🍁 4   🍁 5   🍁 6   🍁 7   🍁 8   🍁 9   🍁 10

"A weed is a plant that has mastered every survival skill except for learning how to grow in rows."
—Doug Larson

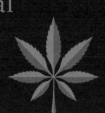

Notes:

Strain Name: _____

Date: _____

Time taken: _____ Time it took to feel effects: _____

Strain Type: □ Sativa □ Indica □ Hybrid □ Not sure

Medium of Consumption: □ Flower □ Edible □ Concentrate □ Other _____

Method: □ Smoke □ Vape □ Ingest □ Other _____

Potency:
(Circle one)

🌿 🌿 🌿 🌿 🌿 🌿 🌿 🌿 🌿 🌿
1 2 3 4 5 6 7 8 9 10

THC % _____ CBD % _____ CBN % _____ Other % _____

Appearance and Taste

Aroma: _____

Color: _____

Flavor Notes: _____

Positive Effects:

□ Creative □ Happy □ Energetic □ Euphoric □ Relaxed □ Talkative

□ Uplifted □ Zen □ Other: _____

Negative Effects:

□ Anxiety □ Cotton mouth □ Couch lock □ Dizziness □ Dry eyes

□ Memory Problems □ Paranoid □ Other: _____

Helps with:

□ General Pain □ Back Pain □ Anxiety □ Depression □ Concentration

□ Sleep Problems □ Other: _____

Would try again?

□ Yes □ No

Overall Rating:
(Circle one)

🌿 🌿 🌿 🌿 🌿 🌿 🌿 🌿 🌿 🌿
1 2 3 4 5 6 7 8 9 10

Notes:

_____

_____

_____

_____

_____

_____

_____

_____

_____

_____

_____

_____

_____

_____

_____

_____

_____

Tip: "Brushing your teeth while high will ensure you're scrubbing 'em for the recommended two minutes. Your dentist will be very happy." (Tanya Chen, *BuzzFeed*)

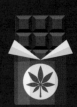

Strain Name: _____

Date: _____

Time taken: _____   Time it took to feel effects: _____

Strain Type: □ Sativa   □ Indica   □ Hybrid   □ Not sure

Medium of Consumption: □ Flower   □ Edible   □ Concentrate   □ Other _____

Method: □ Smoke   □ Vape   □ Ingest   □ Other _____

Potency:
(Circle one)   🍁 🍁 🍁 🍁 🍁 🍁 🍁 🍁 🍁 🍁
          1   2   3   4   5   6   7   8   9   10

THC % _____ CBD % _____ CBN % _____ Other % _____

Appearance and Taste

Aroma: _____

Color: _____

Flavor Notes: _____

Positive Effects:

□ Creative   □ Happy   □ Energetic   □ Euphoric   □ Relaxed   □ Talkative

□ Uplifted   □ Zen   □ Other: _____

Negative Effects:

□ Anxiety   □ Cotton mouth   □ Couch lock   □ Dizziness   □ Dry eyes

□ Memory Problems   □ Paranoid   □ Other: _____

Helps with:

□ General Pain   □ Back Pain   □ Anxiety   □ Depression   □ Concentration

□ Sleep Problems   □ Other: _____

Would try again?

□ Yes   □ No

Overall Rating:
(Circle one)   🍁 🍁 🍁 🍁 🍁 🍁 🍁 🍁 🍁 🍁
          1   2   3   4   5   6   7   8   9   10

> "It really puzzles me to see marijuana connected with narcotics . . . dope and all that crap. It's a thousand times better than whiskey—it's an assistant, a friend." —**Louis Armstrong**

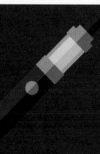

Notes:

Strain Name: _____

Date: _____

Time taken: _____ Time it took to feel effects: _____

Strain Type: ☐ Sativa ☐ Indica ☐ Hybrid ☐ Not sure

Medium of Consumption: ☐ Flower ☐ Edible ☐ Concentrate ☐ Other _____

Method: ☐ Smoke ☐ Vape ☐ Ingest ☐ Other _____

Potency:
(Circle one)

🍁 🍁 🍁 🍁 🍁 🍁 🍁 🍁 🍁 🍁
1　2　3　4　5　6　7　8　9　10

THC % _____ CBD % _____ CBN % _____ Other % _____

Appearance and Taste

Aroma: _____

Color: _____

Flavor Notes: _____

Positive Effects:

☐ Creative ☐ Happy ☐ Energetic ☐ Euphoric ☐ Relaxed ☐ Talkative

☐ Uplifted ☐ Zen ☐ Other: _____

Negative Effects:

☐ Anxiety ☐ Cotton mouth ☐ Couch lock ☐ Dizziness ☐ Dry eyes

☐ Memory Problems ☐ Paranoid ☐ Other: _____

Helps with:

☐ General Pain ☐ Back Pain ☐ Anxiety ☐ Depression ☐ Concentration

☐ Sleep Problems ☐ Other: _____

Would try again?

☐ Yes ☐ No

Overall Rating:
(Circle one)

🍁 🍁 🍁 🍁 🍁 🍁 🍁 🍁 🍁 🍁
1　2　3　4　5　6　7　8　9　10

Notes:

Strain Name: _____

Date: _____

Time taken: _____ Time it took to feel effects: _____

Strain Type: □ Sativa □ Indica □ Hybrid □ Not sure

Medium of Consumption: □ Flower □ Edible □ Concentrate □ Other _____

Method: □ Smoke □ Vape □ Ingest □ Other _____

Potency:
(Circle one)   🍁 🍁 🍁 🍁 🍁 🍁 🍁 🍁 🍁 🍁
               1   2   3   4   5   6   7   8   9   10

THC % _____ CBD % _____ CBN % _____ Other % _____

Appearance and Taste

Aroma: _____

Color: _____

Flavor Notes: _____

Positive Effects:

□ Creative □ Happy □ Energetic □ Euphoric □ Relaxed □ Talkative

□ Uplifted □ Zen □ Other: _____

Negative Effects:

□ Anxiety □ Cotton mouth □ Couch lock □ Dizziness □ Dry eyes

□ Memory Problems □ Paranoid □ Other: _____

Helps with:

□ General Pain □ Back Pain □ Anxiety □ Depression □ Concentration

□ Sleep Problems □ Other: _____

Would try again?

□ Yes □ No

Overall Rating:
(Circle one)   🍁 🍁 🍁 🍁 🍁 🍁 🍁 🍁 🍁 🍁
               1   2   3   4   5   6   7   8   9   10

Notes:

_____

_____

_____

_____

_____

_____

_____

_____

_____

_____

_____

_____

_____

_____

_____

_____

_____

"Its better to cough. Its like, makes you ten times more higher." —Saul Silver, *Pineaple Express*

Strain Name: _____

Date: _____

Time taken: _____ Time it took to feel effects: _____

Strain Type: ☐ Sativa   ☐ Indica   ☐ Hybrid   ☐ Not sure

Medium of Consumption: ☐ Flower   ☐ Edible   ☐ Concentrate   ☐ Other _____

Method: ☐ Smoke   ☐ Vape   ☐ Ingest   ☐ Other _____

Potency:
(Circle one)

    1   2   3   4   5   6   7   8   9   10

THC % _____ CBD % _____ CBN % _____ Other % _____

Appearance and Taste

Aroma: _____

Color: _____

Flavor Notes: _____

Positive Effects:

☐ Creative   ☐ Happy   ☐ Energetic   ☐ Euphoric   ☐ Relaxed   ☐ Talkative

☐ Uplifted   ☐ Zen   ☐ Other: _____

Negative Effects:

☐ Anxiety   ☐ Cotton mouth   ☐ Couch lock   ☐ Dizziness   ☐ Dry eyes

☐ Memory Problems   ☐ Paranoid   ☐ Other: _____

Helps with:

☐ General Pain   ☐ Back Pain   ☐ Anxiety   ☐ Depression   ☐ Concentration

☐ Sleep Problems   ☐ Other: _____

Would try again?

☐ Yes   ☐ No

Overall Rating:
(Circle one)

    1   2   3   4   5   6   7   8   9   10

Tip: For those who vape flowers, don't throw out the finished bud! Save it in a separate container and use it to make edibles (see the recipe for Cannabutter at the end of this book, or use your own recipe).

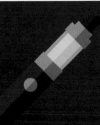

Notes:

Strain Name: _____

Date: _____

Time taken: _____ Time it took to feel effects: _____

Strain Type: □ Sativa □ Indica □ Hybrid □ Not sure

Medium of Consumption: □ Flower □ Edible □ Concentrate □ Other _____

Method: □ Smoke □ Vape □ Ingest □ Other _____

Potency:
(Circle one)

       1   2   3   4   5   6   7   8   9   10

THC % _____ CBD % _____ CBN % _____ Other % _____

Appearance and Taste

Aroma: _____

Color: _____

Flavor Notes: _____

Positive Effects:

□ **Creative** □ **Happy** □ **Energetic** □ **Euphoric** □ **Relaxed** □ **Talkative**

□ **Uplifted** □ **Zen** □ **Other:** _____

Negative Effects:

□ **Anxiety** □ **Cotton mouth** □ **Couch lock** □ **Dizziness** □ **Dry eyes**

□ **Memory Problems** □ **Paranoid** □ **Other:** _____

Helps with:

□ **General Pain** □ **Back Pain** □ **Anxiety** □ **Depression** □ **Concentration**

□ **Sleep Problems** □ **Other:** _____

Would try again?

□ **Yes** □ **No**

Overall Rating:
(Circle one)

       1   2   3   4   5   6   7   8   9   10

> "I tried marijuana once. I did not inhale."
> —Bill Clinton

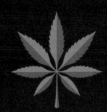

Notes:

Strain Name: _____

Date: _____

Time taken: _____   Time it took to feel effects: _____

Strain Type: ☐ Sativa   ☐ Indica   ☐ Hybrid   ☐ Not sure

Medium of Consumption: ☐ Flower   ☐ Edible   ☐ Concentrate   ☐ Other _____

Method: ☐ Smoke   ☐ Vape   ☐ Ingest   ☐ Other _____

Potency:
(Circle one)

1   2   3   4   5   6   7   8   9   10

THC % _____   CBD % _____   CBN % _____   Other % _____

Appearance and Taste

Aroma: _____

Color: _____

Flavor Notes: _____

Positive Effects:

☐ **Creative**   ☐ **Happy**   ☐ **Energetic**   ☐ **Euphoric**   ☐ **Relaxed**   ☐ **Talkative**

☐ **Uplifted**   ☐ **Zen**   ☐ **Other:** _____

Negative Effects:

☐ **Anxiety**   ☐ **Cotton mouth**   ☐ **Couch lock**   ☐ **Dizziness**   ☐ **Dry eyes**

☐ **Memory Problems**   ☐ **Paranoid**   ☐ **Other:** _____

Helps with:

☐ **General Pain**   ☐ **Back Pain**   ☐ **Anxiety**   ☐ **Depression**   ☐ **Concentration**

☐ **Sleep Problems**   ☐ **Other:** _____

Would try again?

☐ Yes   ☐ No

Overall Rating:
(Circle one)

1   2   3   4   5   6   7   8   9   10

Notes:

_____

_____

_____

_____

_____

_____

_____

_____

_____

_____

_____

_____

_____

_____

_____

_____

Tip: For those Millenial smokers: "Did you know that a Nintendo Gamecube controller is the perfect place to hold your bong head up while you pack it? If you happen to still have a Gamecube, you can use the controller this way to make sure that you're not accidentally dumping out all of your weed."
(Johnny Green, TheWeedBlog.com)

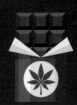

Strain Name: _____

Date: _____

Time taken: _____   Time it took to feel effects: _____

Strain Type: □ Sativa   □ Indica   □ Hybrid   □ Not sure

Medium of Consumption: □ Flower   □ Edible   □ Concentrate   □ Other _____

Method: □ Smoke   □ Vape   □ Ingest   □ Other _____

Potency:
(Circle one)   🍁 🍁 🍁 🍁 🍁 🍁 🍁 🍁 🍁 🍁
                1   2   3   4   5   6   7   8   9   10

THC % _____   CBD % _____   CBN % _____   Other % _____

Appearance and Taste

Aroma: _____

Color: _____

Flavor Notes: _____

Positive Effects:

□ Creative   □ Happy   □ Energetic   □ Euphoric   □ Relaxed   □ Talkative

□ Uplifted   □ Zen   □ Other: _____

Negative Effects:

□ Anxiety   □ Cotton mouth   □ Couch lock   □ Dizziness   □ Dry eyes

□ Memory Problems   □ Paranoid   □ Other: _____

Helps with:

□ General Pain   □ Back Pain   □ Anxiety   □ Depression   □ Concentration

□ Sleep Problems   □ Other: _____

Would try again?

□ Yes   □ No

Overall Rating:
(Circle one)   🍁 🍁 🍁 🍁 🍁 🍁 🍁 🍁 🍁 🍁
                1   2   3   4   5   6   7   8   9   10

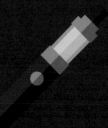

"Weed is from the earth. God put this here for me and you. Take advantage, man. Take advantage."
—Smokey, *Friday*

Notes:

_____

_____

_____

_____

_____

_____

_____

_____

_____

_____

_____

_____

_____

_____

_____

Strain Name: _____

Date: _____

Time taken: _____ Time it took to feel effects: _____

Strain Type: □ Sativa □ Indica □ Hybrid □ Not sure

Medium of Consumption: □ Flower □ Edible □ Concentrate □ Other _____

Method: □ Smoke □ Vape □ Ingest □ Other _____

Potency:
(Circle one)

🍁 🍁 🍁 🍁 🍁 🍁 🍁 🍁 🍁 🍁
1   2   3   4   5   6   7   8   9   10

THC % _____ CBD % _____ CBN % _____ Other % _____

Appearance and Taste

Aroma: _____

Color: _____

Flavor Notes: _____

Positive Effects:

□ **Creative** □ **Happy** □ **Energetic** □ **Euphoric** □ **Relaxed** □ **Talkative**

□ **Uplifted** □ **Zen** □ **Other:** _____

Negative Effects:

□ **Anxiety** □ **Cotton mouth** □ **Couch lock** □ **Dizziness** □ **Dry eyes**

□ **Memory Problems** □ **Paranoid** □ **Other:** _____

Helps with:

□ **General Pain** □ **Back Pain** □ **Anxiety** □ **Depression** □ **Concentration**

□ **Sleep Problems** □ **Other:** _____

Would try again?

□ Yes □ No

Overall Rating:
(Circle one)

🍁 🍁 🍁 🍁 🍁 🍁 🍁 🍁 🍁 🍁
1   2   3   4   5   6   7   8   9   10

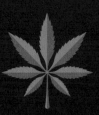

Tip: "Not satisfied with the taste of your edible? Throw it in a smoothie with fruit, Greek yogurt, and your favourite milk substitute." (BluntLifestyle.com)

Notes:

_____

_____

_____

_____

_____

_____

_____

_____

_____

_____

_____

_____

_____

_____

_____

_____

_____

Strain Name: _____

Date: _____

Time taken: _____   Time it took to feel effects: _____

Strain Type: □ Sativa   □ Indica   □ Hybrid   □ Not sure

Medium of Consumption: □ Flower   □ Edible   □ Concentrate   □ Other _____

Method: □ Smoke   □ Vape   □ Ingest   □ Other _____

Potency:
(Circle one)   1   2   3   4   5   6   7   8   9   10

THC % _____   CBD % _____   CBN % _____   Other % _____

Appearance and Taste

Aroma: _____

Color: _____

Flavor Notes: _____

Positive Effects:

□ Creative   □ Happy   □ Energetic   □ Euphoric   □ Relaxed   □ Talkative

□ Uplifted   □ Zen   □ Other: _____

Negative Effects:

□ Anxiety   □ Cotton mouth   □ Couch lock   □ Dizziness   □ Dry eyes

□ Memory Problems   □ Paranoid   □ Other: _____

Helps with:

□ General Pain   □ Back Pain   □ Anxiety   □ Depression   □ Concentration

□ Sleep Problems   □ Other: _____

Would try again?

□ Yes   □ No

Overall Rating:
(Circle one)   1   2   3   4   5   6   7   8   9   10

Notes:

_____

_____

_____

_____

_____

_____

_____

_____

_____

_____

_____

_____

_____

_____

_____

_____

"Marijuana enhances our mind in a way that enables us to take a different perspective from 'high up,' to see and evaluate our own lives and the lives of others in a privileged way. Maybe this euphoric and elevating feeling of the ability to step outside the box and to look at life's patterns from this high perspective is the inspiration behind the slang term 'high' itself."
—Sebastian Marincolo

Strain Name: _____

Date: _____

Time taken: _____ Time it took to feel effects: _____

Strain Type: □ Sativa   □ Indica   □ Hybrid   □ Not sure

Medium of Consumption: □ Flower   □ Edible   □ Concentrate   □ Other _____

Method: □ Smoke   □ Vape   □ Ingest   □ Other _____

Potency:
(Circle one)
1 2 3 4 5 6 7 8 9 10

THC % _____ CBD % _____ CBN % _____ Other % _____

Appearance and Taste

Aroma: _____

Color: _____

Flavor Notes: _____

Positive Effects:

□ **Creative**   □ **Happy**   □ **Energetic**   □ **Euphoric**   □ **Relaxed**   □ **Talkative**

□ **Uplifted**   □ **Zen**   □ **Other:** _____

Negative Effects:

□ **Anxiety**   □ **Cotton mouth**   □ **Couch lock**   □ **Dizziness**   □ **Dry eyes**

□ **Memory Problems**   □ **Paranoid**   □ **Other:** _____

Helps with:

□ **General Pain**   □ **Back Pain**   □ **Anxiety**   □ **Depression**   □ **Concentration**

□ **Sleep Problems**   □ **Other:** _____

Would try again?

□ Yes   □ No

Overall Rating:
(Circle one)
1 2 3 4 5 6 7 8 9 10

Notes:

Strain Name: _____

Date: _____

Time taken: _____ Time it took to feel effects: _____

Strain Type: □ Sativa   □ Indica   □ Hybrid   □ Not sure

Medium of Consumption: □ Flower   □ Edible   □ Concentrate   □ Other _____

Method: □ Smoke   □ Vape   □ Ingest   □ Other _____

Potency:
(Circle one)   🍁   🍁   🍁   🍁   🍁   🍁   🍁   🍁   🍁   🍁
          1   2   3   4   5   6   7   8   9   10

THC % _____ CBD % _____ CBN % _____ Other % _____

Appearance and Taste

Aroma: _____

Color: _____

Flavor Notes: _____

Positive Effects:

□ Creative   □ Happy   □ Energetic   □ Euphoric   □ Relaxed   □ Talkative

□ Uplifted   □ Zen   □ Other: _____

Negative Effects:

□ Anxiety   □ Cotton mouth   □ Couch lock   □ Dizziness   □ Dry eyes

□ Memory Problems   □ Paranoid   □ Other: _____

Helps with:

□ General Pain   □ Back Pain   □ Anxiety   □ Depression   □ Concentration

□ Sleep Problems   □ Other: _____

Would try again?

□ Yes   □ No

Overall Rating:
(Circle one)   🍁   🍁   🍁   🍁   🍁   🍁   🍁   🍁   🍁   🍁
          1   2   3   4   5   6   7   8   9   10

"From a natural stiffness, I melted into a grinning tolerance. Walking on the streets became a high adventure, eating my mother's huge dinners, an opulent entertainment, and playing with my son was side-cracking hilarity. For the first time, life amused me." —Maya Angelou

Notes:

Strain Name: _____

Date: _____

Time taken: _____ Time it took to feel effects: _____

Strain Type: □ Sativa □ Indica □ Hybrid □ Not sure

Medium of Consumption: □ Flower □ Edible □ Concentrate □ Other _____

Method: □ Smoke □ Vape □ Ingest □ Other _____

Potency:
(Circle one)

🍁 🍁 🍁 🍁 🍁 🍁 🍁 🍁 🍁 🍁
1 2 3 4 5 6 7 8 9 10

THC % _____ CBD % _____ CBN % _____ Other % _____

Appearance and Taste

Aroma: _____

Color: _____

Flavor Notes: _____

Positive Effects:

□ **Creative** □ **Happy** □ **Energetic** □ **Euphoric** □ **Relaxed** □ **Talkative**

□ **Uplifted** □ **Zen** □ **Other:** _____

Negative Effects:

□ **Anxiety** □ **Cotton mouth** □ **Couch lock** □ **Dizziness** □ **Dry eyes**

□ **Memory Problems** □ **Paranoid** □ **Other:** _____

Helps with:

□ **General Pain** □ **Back Pain** □ **Anxiety** □ **Depression** □ **Concentration**

□ **Sleep Problems** □ **Other:** _____

Would try again?

□ **Yes** □ **No**

Overall Rating:
(Circle one)

🍁 🍁 🍁 🍁 🍁 🍁 🍁 🍁 🍁 🍁
1 2 3 4 5 6 7 8 9 10

Notes:

_____

_____

_____

_____

_____

_____

_____

_____

_____

_____

_____

_____

_____

_____

_____

Tip: " A little bit of honey will act as glue for a blunt or joint, and it will also make it burn more slowly and evenly." (Alden, World of Weed)

Strain Name: _____

Date: _____

Time taken: _____ Time it took to feel effects: _____

Strain Type: □ Sativa   □ Indica   □ Hybrid   □ Not sure

Medium of Consumption: □ Flower   □ Edible   □ Concentrate   □ Other _____

Method: □ Smoke   □ Vape   □ Ingest   □ Other _____

Potency:
(Circle one)

    1   2   3   4   5   6   7   8   9   10

THC % _____ CBD % _____ CBN % _____ Other % _____

Appearance and Taste

Aroma: _____

Color: _____

Flavor Notes: _____

Positive Effects:

□ Creative   □ Happy   □ Energetic   □ Euphoric   □ Relaxed   □ Talkative

□ Uplifted   □ Zen   □ Other: _____

Negative Effects:

□ Anxiety   □ Cotton mouth   □ Couch lock   □ Dizziness   □ Dry eyes

□ Memory Problems   □ Paranoid   □ Other: _____

Helps with:

□ General Pain   □ Back Pain   □ Anxiety   □ Depression   □ Concentration

□ Sleep Problems   □ Other: _____

Would try again?

□ Yes   □ No

Overall Rating:
(Circle one)

    1   2   3   4   5   6   7   8   9   10

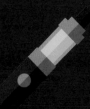

"Even if one doesn't smoke pot one has to see the benefits of decriminalizing it!" —Danny DeVito

Notes:

CANNABUTTER RECIPE

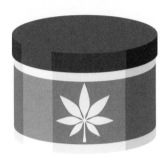

CANNABUTTER

Ingredients:

¼ oz cannabis per stick of butter (1/3 cup cannabis)

1 stick (1/2 cup) unsalted butter

1 ½ cups water

Cheese cloth

Tupperware container

Step-by-Step

1. In a saucepan, pour 1 ½ cups water and ground cannabis.

2. Simmer on low heat, stirring frequently.

3. Once water/cannabis are heated (there will be movement in the water from small bubbles), place stick of butter in saucepan.

4. Let butter/water/cannabis mixture simmer on low heat for 2 to 3 hours, stirring every 10 to 15 minutes.

5. While the mixture is simmering, grab a Tupperware container and place cheesecloth on top, securing with a rubberband. Note: using at least two to three

layers of cheese cloth, so as to remove bit of cannabis remaining that only one layer of cloth would not catch.

6. After the mixture has been simmering for 2 to 3 hours (bud will become very dark and start to sink to the bottom of the saucepan), pour the mixture into the prepared Tupperware container.

7. Remove cheese cloth from Tupperware container so that all of the cannabis is inside the cloth.

8. Drain the liquid from the cannabis by squeezing the bag of soggy bud in between two flat surfaces to get the rest of the liquid out and into the tupperware.

9. Put the lid on the Tupperware and let the liquid sit in the fridge for 3 to 4 hours, or until all the butter has solidified on top of the wter (best to do overnight or while you have something to do during the day). Note: If you feel it to be necessary, you can melt your butter and strain it again to get out any additional impurities that may not have been caught the first time. Then continue the rest of this step.

10. Make any recipe (that includes butter, of course) as you would normally, but instead spice it up with your "special butter."

Note: It will take 30 or more minutes to take effect, so do *not* eat more than one (or two) of your baked goodies before you know how your body reacts.

GLOSSARY OF TERMS

This glossary originates from *The Art of Marijuana Etiquette: A Sophisticated Guide to the High Life* by Andrew Ward.

Bhang: An edible from India, used traditionally during the spring Holi festival.

BHO: Butane-based hash oil extraction.

Blaze: To smoke cannabis.

Blunt: A type of marijuana cigarette made famous by the Phillies Blunts brands of cigars.

Blunt ride: The act of driving around while smoking a blunt or other type of marijuana cigarette.

Bong: A water pipe for smoking, which employs a downstem, a connected bowl, and water to produce the smoke.

Bowl: The part of a pipe where the ground cannabis is placed for smoking.

Bubbler: A water pipe similar to a *Bong*, except that it is typically hand-held.

Bud: A term for marijuana with no clear origin.

Budtender: A dispensary employee tasked with assisting the customer during their sales experience.

Cannabidiol (CBD): A non-intoxicating cannabinoid with various reported medicinal benefits, becoming very popular among consumers in recent years.

Cannabinoids: Naturally occurring cannabinoids found in the cannabis sativa plant, each providing varying effects when consumed.

Cannabis intoxication: When a person consumes too much cannabis, leading them to experience the adverse associated effects.

Cannabis shakes: A relatively harmless phenomenon that occurs when a person consumes too much marijuana.

Cashed: The end of a session. Applies to bowls down to the resinous black bits. Or, the tail end of marijuana cigarette.

Caviar: *Nugs* dipped in oil extracts and rolled in *kief* for additional potency. Some may claim the process does not involve kief. Also known as "Moon Rocks."

Cheeba: A term for marijuana that, depending on the region, may also refer to heroin.

Chillum Pipe: A small, straight or coned device used for smoking cannabis. Traditionally made from clay, though modern creations include ceramic, wood and metal.

Choom: A Hawaiian term for smoking. Made famous by former US president Barack Obama's and his high school smoking buddies, known as the "Choom Gang."

Chronic: Top-quality marijuana. Made famous by Dr. Dre's 1992 album *The Chronic*.

Churro: Spanish for a rolled marijuana joint or cigarette.

Circle: A smoke circle.

Clone: Genetic copy of the mother plant, used instead of growing with seeds.

Concentrates: Cannabis products created from extracted oils from the plant. Also known as an *extract*.

Corssfaded: The feeling and effects brought on by excessive consumption of marijuana and alcohol.

Dab Rig: A pipe used for vaporizing concentrates. Often referred to as a *rig*.

Dagga: South African slang for marijuana stemming from the Khoi word *dacha*.

Dank: High-quality pot describing sticky, green, pungent nugs, often rich in skunky aromas.

Dealer: Your illegal cannabis delivery person or service. *See Plug*

Devil's Lettuce: A nineteenth-century term for cannabis used as propaganda, now used in a comical sense.

Dime Bag: A $10 bag of pot that usually contains a half to one full gram.

Dispensary: A legal storefront where cannabis is sold.

Doobie: American slang for a marijuana cigarette. Origins are uncertain, but likely connect to the rock band The Doobie Brothers.

Dugout: A two-chamber wooden box that holds ground cannabis and a chillum. The pipe is used for retrieving the cannabis from the chamber for smoking. Often referred to as a One Hitter.

Edible: Food or drinks infused with cannabis.

Erba: Italian slang for marijuana.

Extract: *See Concentrate*

Extraction: The process by which oils, cannabinoids and terpenes are taken from the plant.

Faso: Argentine term for marijuana cigarette.

Flavonoids: A phytonutrient found in cannabis and just about every fruit or vegetable. One of the many compounds believed to be essential in creating the unique effects in each cannabis strain.

Flower: General term for marijuana.

Ganja: A common term for cannabis stemming from Hindi culture, rather than Rastafarian where it is often misattributed.

Grass: English slang for marijuana most popular during the 1960s and 1970s. Known as Gras in other languages..

Grinder: A multi-chamber tool used to break apart nugs into smaller pieces for smoking in a variety of devices.

Heads: The number of people consuming pot in a group.

Hierba (Yerba): Spanish for grass.

Hybrid: The result of breeding two or more plants together, aiming to inherit the best traits of each strain.

Hydroponic: A form of soilless cultivation using suspended roots and direct nutrient application.

Indica: Cannabis term used to classify strains which tend to induce relaxing, calming effects. Commonly known as putting people "In da couch" when consumed.

Indoor: Cannabis that was grown in an artificial grow setting.

Joint: Marijuana cigarette made using thin rolling papers.

J's: Joints.

Kief: Dried resin of the cannabis plant. Also known as *hash*.

Loud: Pungent, potent marijuana.

Maja: Swedish slang for marijuana.

Marijuana cigarette: A more formal term for a joint, blunt, or spliff.

Mary Jane: English slang for pot, likely originating from the Spanish term *marijuana*.

Match: Throwing in an equal amount of pot as other contributors in the circle.

Medical: Cannabis and its products made for patients with medical needs.

Moon Rocks: *See Caviar*

Mota: Mexican slang for marijuana.

Mother Plant: The source plant growers use for cloning purposes.

Munchies: Food cravings brought on by cannabis consumption.

Nickel Bag: A $5 bag of pot that tends to contain one quarter of a gram of pot.

Nugs: Cannabis buds, often referring to higher quality marijuana.

OGs: Sometimes referred to as "legacy cannabis" members, the OGs are the originators that helped take the market from the outlaw days to what it is today. In some cases, OGs continue to fight the system and refuse to join the legal market.

One Hitter: *See Dugout*

Outdoor: Cannabis that was grown in natural settings, exposed to sunlight and natural settings.

Plant profile: The makeup of a strain, including its potency, terpenes, cannabinoids, and flavinoids.

Plug: A source for what you need. In cannabis, relating to your dealer or delivery service.

Porro: Spanish slang for *joint*.

Pot: A common slang term for marijuana with unclear origins.

Potency: A term used to describe the percentage of a compound found in the cannabis product, often referring to THC or CBD.

Pre-roll: A joint prepared prior to purchasing.

Public Consumption: The legal practice of getting high in public spaces. *See Lowell Cafe/the Cannabis Cafe*

Puff: English slang for marijuana, used primarily in England.

Reefer: A common slang term for marijuana with uncertain origins.

Run: The act of going out and buying cannabis. Can be used to describe other tasks as well, often linked to getting snacks (Snack Run).

Sativa: Cannabis term used to classify strains which tend to induce uplifting, energetic effects.

SHO: Hash oil extraction using natural elements rather than solvents.

Shotgun: A potent technique used when a person blows smoke into the mouth of another person in the circle.

Sketchy: A suspicious person. In pot terms, someone who is unreliable with their time, money or is creepy in general.

Smoke out: To get someone high on your supply without asking for anything in return.

Stoned: The feeling associated with consuming large amounts of marijuana.

Strain: A term used to describe the various types of cannabis varieties created. The term has no scientific connection, often interchanged with terms like *cultivar*.

Terpenes: Organic compounds that, when in cannabis, shape the strain's aromatic and flavor profile, as well as its effects.

Tincture: Liquid cannabis extract produced using alcohol or glycerin, often flavored and packaged with a dropper for dosing.

Torch: A propane or butane lighter used to hear a dab rig's nail.

Trichome: The oily, sticky hairs found on the cannabis plant, holding the flower's cannabinoids and terpenes.

Twist it up: The twisting technique performed at the end of a joint rolling session.

Vape: The act of inhaling on a vaporizer, colloquially used by some to describe the battery and its cartridge, as well.

Vape Cartridge: A container filled with extracted cannabis oil used for vaping.

Wiet: Dutch word for *weed*.

Additional Notes:

Additional Notes:

Additional Notes:

Additional Notes:

Additional Notes:

Additional Notes:

Additional Notes:

Additional Notes:

THE ART OF
MARIJUANA
ETIQUETTE

A SOPHISTICATED GUIDE
TO THE HIGH LIFE

❋ ANDREW WARD ❋

The Art of Marijuana Etiquette
A Sophisticated Guide to the High Life
by Andrew Ward

When it comes to cannabis, there are numerous unspoken rules that users take very seriously. Whether we're talking about puff, puff, pass or supplying your own munchies, the marijuana community has always tried to keep etiquette as a staple of the lifestyle. Now, from one stoner to another, *The Art of Marijuana Etiquette* will guide you through all phases of weed life so you can enjoy the highest quality hydroponic without being disrespectful to those around you. Some key lessons include:

· Understanding the language and terminology

· Step-by-step details on how to roll

· Tips and tricks to improve your smoking session

· How to prepare for a visit to legal dispensaries

· And much more.

As the negative connotation of marijuana begins to dissipate, there will be more people partaking than ever. That's why noted journalist Andrew Ward has sat down with those in the marijuana community to find out what they find the most important lessons to share, so that veteran and amateur smokers can get the most out of this incredible plant. Having this handy guide to teach you in the ways of weed will make sure that you can continue the proud tradition of respect among stoners, while also educating those joining the party on how to carry themselves. Respect is key, and the more you understand about how to enjoy and medicate with cannabis, the better we will all be.

$15.99 Paperback · ISBN 978-1-5107-5465-2